Monitoring Children's Health:

Key Indicators

Second Edition

American Public Health Association
1015 Fifteenth Street, NW
Washington, DC 20005

William H. McBeath, MD, MPH, Executive Director

The opinions expressed in this publication are the authors' and do not necessarily represent the views or official policies of the Association.

Printed and bound in the United States of America.

Design: Dan Winter, Emerson Braxton & Co., Silver Spring, MD
Typesetting: Athens Enterprises, Ltd., Ijamsville, MD
Printing and Binding: St. Mary's Press, Hollywood, MD

ISBN 0–87553–162–8

3M4/89

Monitoring Children's Health: Key Indicators

Second Edition

C. ARDEN MILLER
AMY FINE
SHARON ADAMS-TAYLOR

American Public Health Association
1015 Fifteenth Street, NW
Washington, DC 20005

Acknowledgments

This work, including the second edition, is a product of the Child Health Outcomes Project, Department of Maternal and Child Health, School of Public Health, University of North Carolina. The project obtained support from many sources; the most substantial support was from the Ford Foundation. The authors are grateful to Oscar Harkavy, Chief Program Officer for the Ford Foundation, for his encouragement and support.

Table of Contents

Preface to the Second Edition

The first edition of this book was prepared in the context of dramatic changes in national health policies. New policies implemented with the Reagan administration promoted private and competitive initiatives for the provision of health services and scaled back government's role. Insofar as government retained responsibility for the protection of health, this responsibility was pushed toward state and local levels. Federal government not only reduced its financing for preventive health services, but diminished the identification of priorities that accompany categorical financing. For many programs, including income transfers, payments for medical care, and nutrition for school children, eligibility was restricted and benefits were reduced.

All of these changes were made in the midst of reassurances that no one would be hurt. To many people, the reassurances appeared both hollow and ominous. The condition of children and the programs that benefited them had never been better than marginal. Constructive endeavors that had been limited in their effectiveness by small budgets and rising inflation were constrained even more.

Along with other cutbacks, official data-gathering and reporting systems were reduced, making the careful monitoring of trends in child health exceedingly difficult. Requirements were weakened for the states to report on changes in scope of services and health trends of populations dependent on federally financed health programs. Unlike the previous categorical health care programs, the new block grants carried no obligation for evaluation or reporting of services.

The response to these changes was impressive: Advocacy organizations, professional associations, research projects, and state health and welfare departments mobilized to gather data and issue reports on trends in maternal and child health. The Child Health Outcomes Project of the University of North Carolina at one time identified more than 50 endeavors of more than narrowly local interest attempting to report on the condition of the nation's children. All of these endeavors were aimed at garnering current data to inform considerations of public policy as it affects children's health. The first edition of this book was designed to assist these endeavors by identifying policy-relevant indicators, promoting consistency of their definition, identifying data sources, and suggesting the relevance of these indicators to public policy.

Circumstances are changing. The weight of evidence confirms that children have indeed suffered under recent policies. Areas showing worsening trends, sometimes for large vulnerable population subgroups, include utilization of prenatal care, rates of low birth weight and infant mortality, immunization status, and number of cases of child abuse and neglect. For other indicators, data sources have been so diminished that careful monitoring cannot be done or must be delayed over a long time span. These circumstances pertain to iron deficiency anemia, growth stunting, lead poisoning, immunizations, and child abuse.

The most substantial change is an increase in the proportion of children living in poverty. Even as unemployment rates have fallen and some other important measures of the nation's economic vigor have improved, more than one in five children lives in poverty-level households. For minority children and those in single-parent families, the poverty rate is much higher. Along with this ominous trend, new evidence has been marshalled on the great damage done to children because they are poor and, as a consequence in our society, deprived of many essential services and supports.

Many voices have been raised in response to these circumstances. New, carefully documented formulations of children's health and family policy are impressive not only for their passion but for their substance. Shallow sentimentality, once prevalent and perhaps thought to be sufficient for promoting maternal and child health, has given way to carefully fortified logic that identifies the salient problems and points the way to their resolution. Especially noteworthy are the annual publications from the Children's Defense Fund and the recent report from the Office of Technology Assessment, and Schorr's upbeat call to national action in her new book, *Within Our Reach, Breaking the Cycle of Disadvantage* (Doubleday, New York, 1988). This book makes the case for government's role in protecting children and identifies the limitations of market economy as a suitable substitute.

The public conscience is being mobilized on behalf of children in ways reminiscent of the surge of concern that preceded the social reforms in the first two decades of this century around issues of child labor and infant abandonment. The ways of reform for the years ahead are not yet self-evident, but one thing is clear. Reform will be benefited by good data. This book has been revised and its data made current in the hope that it will be useful to conscientious people who will strive to improve maternal and child health policies and programs in the years ahead.

Since publication of the first edition, other valuable reviews of trends in child health have been published, each of which complements the data in this text. Readers are urged to consult the following:
- Office of Technology Assessment. Healthy children, investing in the future. Washington, DC: Congress of the U.S., 1987.

- Office of Disease Prevention and Health Promotion. Disease prevention health promotion: the facts. Palo Alto, CA: U.S. Public Health Service, U.S. Department of Health and Human Services, 1988.
- U.S. House of Representatives, Select Committee on Children, Youth, and Families. U.S. children and their families: current conditions and recent trends. Washington, DC: U.S. House of Representatives, 100th Congress, 1987.
- Children's Defense Fund. The health of America's children. MCH Data Book, Washington, DC: CDF, 1988.
- Children's Defense Fund. A children's defense budget, FY1989. Washington, DC: CDF, 1988.

CHAPTER 1

Introduction

The social supports and health services available for children are exceedingly variable from one part of the country to another and from one population subgroup to another. Income and nutritional supplementation for children, as well as access to health care, fluctuate over time as different public policies prevail, guided by an inconstant perception of their effectiveness and feasibility. These changing circumstances prompt concern about their impact on the health of children.

Children are known to be resilient and adaptable. Can they adjust to their changing environments and continue to develop in ways that are promising for their own prospects and encouraging for society's future? Children are also known to be vulnerable and easily damaged by social, psychic, and physical traumas or neglect. This vulnerability is especially great for children who are not well nurtured in the fullest sense of that concept. If children are blighted by failures to meet their needs, what are the long- and short-term costs to society? What interventions are most substantially linked to improved health for children? What is society's responsibility to assist families in the care of children? What social values, regardless of financial costs, need to be considered and protected?

Answers to many of these questions depend on a better understanding of trends in the health of children and the circumstances that influence these trends. This book is designed to enhance such understanding.

The Relationship Between Data Gathering and Public Policy

A reciprocal, interactive relationship has always existed between data gathering and public policy. Prevailing policies have generated the need for certain kinds of data; conversely, the reported findings have been fed into the dynamics of policy development as justification for modifications in service interventions and changes in the resources required to sustain them.

Health policy may be regarded as the aggregate of principles or themes that prevail in the ways society distributes its resources and power as they relate to the determinants of a population's state of health. "Resources," of course, refers to goods and money; "power" refers to accreditations, licensures, and entitlements as they relate to health care. In this country the ways these benefactions are distributed are not fixed, but are negotiated among competing interest groups. Powerful players in this dynamic include the medical profession, hospitals, insurance companies, health industry entrepreneurs, and, in recent years, the major sources of financing for medical care, government and large employers.

The health of children is not necessarily well served by a negotiated health policy, unless their interests are protected either by government regulation or by advocacy groups that participate in the negotiating process. Both of these alternatives require access to information predictive of children's needs.

Certain discernible themes have prevailed at different times in recent history, and these themes have had an important interaction with the kinds of data that were regarded as important. Considerations of the biological and medical determinants of health have usually dominated health policy, bringing many advantages to American medicine in the form of advanced technology. Problems regarding how access to this technology can be equitably distributed have not been resolved. Tensions surround a realization that medical care in the United States is rationed, largely on the basis of ability to pay for it. Medical domination of health policy fosters neglect of other domains, such as those concerned with education, the environment, and social supports. In matters of health policy we behave as if we seek medical answers to social problems, even at great expense, rather than engaging in social reforms that might have a more meaningful impact on health status.

The major determinants of favorable maternal and child health status relate to quality-of-life issues: nurture, social supports, nutrition, housing, and education. Although the interlocking relationships between social and biological determinants of good health have been known for many years, prevailing health policy has not generally been responsive to these complex linkages.

A simple schematic is often used to clarify the dynamics that are invoked for administering human support services: Resources (e.g., personnel and facilities) are used in certain ways (processes) to yield identifiable outcomes:

Resources → Processes → Outcomes

This diagram can be elaborated with branches and feedbacks, but its simple form helps characterize some dominant themes of health policy.

During the 1950s and 1960s, national health policy featured an acknowledged responsibility for government to provide the resources judged to be essential for health care. Training health workers, constructing hospitals, and developing medical technology were all judged to be public responsibilities. Justifications were found in abundant data that were generated around such measures as physician-to-population ratios, distribution of hospital beds, and access to appropriate diagnostic and treatment services. Improvements in these measures were presumed to be associated with improved health or some other social good, without ever defining these benefits precisely.

Later in the 1960s and in the 1970s, attention was focused on the processes by which health care resources are used. Duplications and gaps in the distribution of services were recognized as important problems. Efforts to plan and in some measure to regulate the allocation of resources (e.g., the National Health Service Corps and certificates of need for hospital construction) became important features of health policy. Certain kinds of provider systems and methods for payment were promoted to improve care for the underserved (e.g., neighborhood health centers and Medicaid) and to promote preventive services and to reduce costs (e.g., health maintenance organizations and use of physicians' assistants and nurse practitioners). Studies that were presumed to have special relevance to policy featured data on processes: distribution, cost of health services, and financing systems. Data on utilization of services, particularly among population subgroups, gained new importance. Narrowing the gap in the number of physician visits between poor and nonpoor children was regarded as an important indicator of success for the new prevailing health policies.

Interest has always been high in survival data, such as age-specific mortality rates, including infant mortality, and survival rates from dread diseases. These data have sometimes been used to influence resource allocations for targeted research or for disease-specific screening, diagnostic, and treatment services. For example, in the 1920s, the nation's comparatively high maternal mortality rate prompted passage of the Sheppard-Towner Act, which distributed federal funds to the states in support of maternal and child health services. In the 1960s, concern over high infant mortality rates, coupled with an effort to prevent some forms of mental retardation, stimulated special maternal and child health service projects in selected areas. Using similar justifications, special grants were also made to some of the poorest states to achieve improved pregnancy outcomes. These initiatives represented a departure from the prevailing policy themes: Each initiative was designed to achieve some stated health status objective, or outcome, measurable in terms of human survival or well-being.

The greatest impetus for using outcome data, in addition to data on resources and processes, came in the late 1970s and early 1980s with growing concern about high governmental expenditures for health care. This concern fostered an expectation that resource inputs and the ways in which resources were used should be held accountable. Cost-benefit analysis and evaluations of program effectiveness became urgent. These procedures required that program benefits and objectives be well defined. Few of the programs had been established with an obligation for achieving precisely defined objectives or for collecting data sufficient for evaluating cost-effectiveness. These difficulties enabled the Reagan administration, in the major budget reductions of 1981, to reduce support for many health related services while claiming that no evidence could be marshalled to demonstrate that people would suffer as a consequence of the reduction.

Attention to measurable health status outcomes and risks thus achieved new prominence in analysis of health policy. New kinds of data were required. In the face of reduced monitoring and reporting at the federal level, new initiatives for gathering, analyzing, and reporting policy-relevant data in a timely fashion became urgent at the state and community levels. New interest focused on how the task could be done. Voluntary health advocacy groups, as well as the official health agencies of state and local governments, addressed the need for health risk or outcome data for their constituent populations.

After passage of the Omnibus Budget Reconciliation Act of 1981, federal funding for social support and health service programs was reduced, and responsibility for administering many of the programs shifted from the federal to the state level of government. The federal administration offered assurances that no one would be seriously hurt by these changes; a safety net was in place to protect truly needy people from serious harm. The safety net was presumed to consist of the residual supportive programs, but no new monitoring efforts were put in place to measure the safety net's adequacy. On the contrary, many centralized reporting systems were diminished; as new responsibilities for implementation of programs were shifted to the states, requirements for reporting to federal agencies were greatly reduced. State and local governments, as well as many concerned voluntary agencies, began evaluating the impact of these policy and program changes on vulnerable populations.

Even in previous administrations, measurement of these trends had been regularly done in only a sketchy way. Some useful sources of information are national census data; the National Health and Nutrition Examination Survey (NHANES), the National Health Interview Survey (NHIS), and the monthly reporting of provisional data on births and deaths, all by the National Center for Health Statistics (NCHS); the Food Consumption Survey of the Department of Agriculture; and various reports, as on immunizations and lead poisoning, by the Centers for Disease Control. Abundant as the data sources seem to be, however, they all suffer serious shortcomings for monitoring children's health.[14] The most serious shortcoming of all is tardiness of reporting. Many of the reports are issued many years after the events for which an evaluation of impact is sought. Consequently, health and social programs are begun, modified, or terminated based on only partially informed judgments of their effectiveness.

Large amounts of potentially useful data are collected and never interpreted in the context of the policy implications. The rigor of scientific inquiry inveighs against interpretations that risk speculation on the applicability of research findings. A different discipline guides policy makers. They must allocate resources, set priorities, and regulate procedures, acting on whatever data are available, and yielding to the force of value judgments that associate with the greatest powers of negotiation. In this fluid situation, the hope is strong that values which are promoted contrary to available evidence will not endure for long.

Good data and public policy are natural allies, but they have sometimes gone their separate ways, often with unhappy consequences. For example, many states have rescinded laws requiring motorcyclists to wear helmets or motorists to use seat belts despite overwhelming evidence of their protective value. In these instances arguments in favor of personal freedoms have taken precedence over data on death, disability, and the related societal expense. Another example relates to cigarette smoking. Evidence that deaths, disability, and associated great costs for medical care are attributable to cigarette smoking is extensive, yet the federal government continues to subsidize tobacco growers. Value judgments rooted in data on the economic interests of tobacco-growing areas are an important ingredient of this public policy. Another example relates to the work of midwives and nurse practitioners. Despite abundant data on the many advantages, including improved access and reduced cost, associated with these providers, no substantial provision has been made to use them.

Concern for Child Health Outcomes

The University of North Carolina Child Health Outcomes Project was begun in 1982 in the belief that access to sound data interpreted in a timely fashion could improve advocacy and the public policies that emerge from it. The project began with the conviction that measures of health outcomes, or measures of process interventions clearly linked to identifiable outcomes, should receive increased attention in policy formulation and program accountability. Otherwise the distribution of resources and development of programs, even though touted in the name of children's health, can become distorted to serve many interests far afield from the expressed goal.

Emphasis on outcome objectives as the organizing principle of public policy shows promise for rationalizing the allocation of resources and the planning of services. If outcome objectives are clearly identified, the antecedent interventions, and the resources required to implement them, must be justified in terms of the evidence that links them to the objectives. In this manner, both the resources and the interventions can be held accountable by measuring progress toward achieving the outcome objectives. This chain of logic carries the further advantage of demedicalizing approaches to improve health. All interventions, including those in the arenas of education and social welfare, come under consideration for evaluating their contributions toward achieving agreed-upon outcomes. Agreements on desirable and feasible outcomes among human support agencies could form a new basis for collaboration in the bureaucratic infrastructure.

Relation to Other Endeavors

Thinking about outcome objectives is not new to people in public health. The objectives for *Model Standards for Community Preventive Health Services*[2] and those for the program known as *Promoting Health/Preventing Disease: Objectives for the Nation*[8] represent this same direction of thought. A collaboration involving the Centers for Disease Control (CDC) of the U.S. Public Health Service (PHS) and several national health organizations produced the *Model Standards for Community Preventive Health Services* in August 1979. These standards departed from previous approaches by stressing outcome and process objectives and avoiding standards for resource inputs, or for their structural organization. The report acknowledged that the objectives might be achieved in different ways according to local circumstances and that local discretion should be preserved for promoting the most appropriate local strategies. The objectives were organized into 33 traditional public health categorical programs. These standards are now available in the 1985 revised edition.[1] An increasing number of state and local public health agencies are making use of the model standards as the organizing principle for community services.

Similar concepts but different organizational principles were incorporated into *Promoting Health/Preventing Disease: Objectives for the Nation,* developed by the Public Health Service and published in the fall of 1980.[8] Unlike the model standards, these objectives were designed not for the community, but for the nation at large. A categorical approach was abandoned in favor of three broadly defined endeavors: preventive health services, health protection, and health promotion. The objectives within these endeavors were clustered, when possible, according to age-specific groupings. The objectives emphasized outcomes and were substantially the same as the model standards. This duplication can be attributed in part to the circumstance that many of the same experts worked on both projects, and in larger part to the limitations of current understandings concerning well-documented health status indicators.

The formulation of measurable national health objectives, begun in the Carter administration, survived throughout two Reagan administrations, but the cause did not flourish. Survival of the effort is noteworthy in the midst of ideologies strongly oriented toward priorities set by market economics rather than by social planners. Perhaps, even in the midst of conservative ideologies, management by objective found some favor.

The nation's progress toward achieving the 1990 Objectives in maternal and child health has been disappointing; many objectives will not be realized. Hearings were held in 1988 on reformulation of the objectives for the year 2000. The presented evidence supported retaining and reinforcing the objectives and even expanding them into other areas of endeavor. No voices claimed that the objectives were inappropriate or undesirable. With minor exceptions the targets were deemed feasible, and more intense effort was urged to achieve them.

Dr. J. Michael McGinnis has thoughtfully analyzed the conceptual underpinnings for setting national health objectives.[6] His report described the objectives and the process by which they were selected, relating the entire endeavor to experience with management by objective. He made no claim that consideration of measurable outcome objectives yet drives health policy in the United States, but it is having an impact. A public conscience is stirring, for example, around such issues as high infant mortality rates and childbearing by young teenagers.

Block grants and contracts with insurance companies or other major providers could be written in such a way as to require compliance with uniform national standards, based on the model standards for community preventive health services. Progress toward meeting standards based on outcome objectives could be used as an instrument of accountability for success in meeting the terms of public financing. Such steps might go a long way toward defining and maintaining priorities consistently and equitably in all parts of the country and for all population subgroups.

These speculations require amplification on two points. The first acknowledges that the use of outcome measures cannot be purist. Some processes (e.g., family planning) have greater public health utility for purposes of public policy than the outcomes to which the processes are strongly linked. For example, measuring the extent to which newborn babies are unwanted is possible, but the procedures for doing so are cumbersome. Utilization rates of contraception by sexually active couples have greater utility for consideration of public policy.

A second amplification addresses the complex interplay of public, private, and voluntary endeavors that contribute to improved health for children. These endeavors can relate to each other most productively if they share a sense of purpose. Focusing their efforts on agreed-upon outcome measures would be helpful. Those of us working in public health are dedicated to an additional cause: an official agency operational at local levels, concerned with monitoring health status, and able to offer all children, by contract or by direct service, the basic supports that ad hoc arrangements may not consistently address.

Selection of Indicators

This book attempts to strengthen the foundation of solid data on which sound policy in matters of children's health can be built. Twelve indicators of child health are fully described, and data sources are identified. For each indicator the policy implications are reviewed. This analysis identifies past experience and best judgments about the programmatic initiatives that hold promise for improving health status as measured by the indicators.

The child health indicators presented here were selected, after extensive consultations, as representative of child health problems that can, with the present state of knowledge, be prevented or reduced in the population and about which data are relatively easy to obtain. Data based on these indicators are intended to illuminate the extent to which social policy in general, and health services in particular, has been effectively directed to meet child health needs. Each of the indicators was judged salient to the interests and concerns of the public and policy makers.

The indicators are offered as a starting point for gathering data on child health. They are not intended to be a complete list of all the important child health outcomes and risks that can be measured. The following questions guided the choice of each indicator:

- Is it widely regarded by experts in the field as reflecting important health or policy concerns?
- Is it understandable to and considered significant by the public and policy makers?
- Can data on the indicator be obtained relatively easily?
- Does it relate to a disease, condition, or cause of death that could be prevented or greatly reduced through known and available interventions?

Several other considerations influenced this list. Two process measures, immunization and prenatal care, are included because they are widely regarded as having a consistent influence on health status or on risk, are readily measured, and represent a policy emphasis that is more timely than the related health outcomes. For example, waiting for an outbreak of poliomyelitis (the outcome) would be poor health practice in a population known to have low immunization rates (the process or risk assessment). A different motivation relates to prenatal care. It is by no means the perfect surrogate for outcome measures such as birth weight or infant mortality, but its association with these measures is strong for high-risk populations, and measuring prenatal care is feasible for populations too small for meaningful analysis of the outcomes.

The list of indicators is intended to permit selective application appropriate for population bases of different size, and to monitoring groups of different sophistication and interest. Strategies need to be selected and designed in ways that are specific to the circumstances of different communities and subpopulations. The criterion that data be readily available does not preclude use of surveys or special studies, if procedures are relatively simple and can be conveniently described and carried out.

Roads Not Taken

All of the measures presented in this book are well-recognized indicators for physical health, risk, and survival. Psychosocial measures and indicators for more subtle aspects of good health are not included. Such indicators might include the following:

- failure to thrive,
- multiple foster home placements,
- days missed from school,
- disabling conditions,
- perceptual disorders (corrected and uncorrected),
- learning disability,
- school failures or dropouts,
- inappropriate or specialized school placements,
- behavioral disturbances,
- involvement in violent crime,
- substance abuse, and
- a regular source of medical care.

These measures may have great utility for research or for well-controlled evaluations. For example, some of the indicators have been useful for measuring the long-range adjustments after early enriched day care, such as Head Start. For widespread use by different monitoring groups, however, the indicators suffer from lack of precision and consistency of definition. For many of the indicators, no reliable data sources are readily available and collecting primary data requires elaborate procedures. For others, the policy implications are by no means clear. For example, on the surface, days missed from school would appear to be a useful indicator of health status for school-aged children. This turns out not to be the case. The quality of the school may have a greater impact than students' health on attendance. Also, the nature of the family and home are important determinants. For some healthy children, staying out of school to assist with family needs may represent a higher order of adjustment than attending school.

Many of the phychosocial indicators that are not described in this report will nonetheless find important application, most often under well-controlled circumstances that do not depend on baseline standards and that involve comparisons between one group and a similar control group. These conditions constrain the use of many indicators, limiting them to sophisticated and expensive special purposes. The set of indicators fully described here is intended to highlight the most basic kinds of information needed for making major decisions that will shape child health policy for the next decade.

Another method for monitoring health invokes the use of sentinel events—that is, events (disease, disability, or untimely death) that should never happen or should happen only rarely. The occurrence of even one of these events, even without complete data on the population base, signals that something is seriously remiss and that remedial measures are indicated. Examples of such sentinel events include a case of diphtheria, a septic abortion, or cancer of the cervix diagnosed in advanced states. As explained by Rutstein et al.,

> The chain of responsibility to prevent the occurrence of any unnecessary disease, disability, or untimely death may be long and complex. The failure of any single link may precipitate an unnecessary, undesirable health event. Thus, the unnecessary case of diphtheria, measles, or poliomyelitis may be the responsibility of the state legislature that neglected to appropriate the needed funds, the health officer who did not implement the program, the medical society that opposed community clinics, the physician who did not immunize his patient, the religious views of the family, or the mother who didn't bother to take her baby for immunization.[11]

This formulation gives appropriate emphasis to the importance of community diagnosis and policy analysis as companion efforts to monitoring health status. A case of diphtheria or data on immunization rates or on infant mortality may identify the presence of a serious problem; the antecedent circumstances that contribute to the problem and the most appropriate remedial measures for correcting it will differ substantially from one population subgroup or one community to another.

Some sentinel events of special importance to child health care are these:

- measles,
- tetanus,
- diphtheria,
- poliomyelitis,
- congenital syphilis,
- mental retardation due to phenylketonuria or hypothyroidism,
- vitamin D deficient rickets, and
- diarrheal death.

In addition, homelessness can now join the list of sentinel events of importance to children. It once was a problem reserved for derelicts and the mentally ill, but now entire families are homeless. In some communities, as many as a third of homeless people may be children. Their plight indicates a breakdown of community services that support vulnerable people.

Emphasis on these and other outcome measures for monitoring child health broadens the scope of considerations for appropriate interventions. Health problems may thus become demedicalized as effective preventive measures become well documented in the domains of education, nutrition, social welfare, or environmental protection. As with all indicators, they suggest that attention be directed toward a broad range of issues, including access to contraception, family health education, recreation, and job opportunities.

This book updates information about the same 12 indicators that were included in the earlier edition. Consideration was given also to other indicators, including reported cases of rheumatic fever, acquired immunodeficiency syndrome (AIDS) infection in children, and poverty rates.

Rheumatic Fever

Attack rates of acute rheumatic fever have been used successfully to compare the effectiveness of early diagnosis and treatment under different health care systems. Rheumatic fever is known to occur as a complication of inadequately treated streptococcal infections. Monitoring the rates of the complication among different groups of children therefore can be a device for measuring the relative adequacy of their different forms of medical care.

Within recent years a surge has occurred in the number of reported cases of rheumatic fever. This increase appears to be associated with changes in the type and virulence of the streptococcus organism, and not with the adequacy of treatment.[5] The policy significance of this development has acquired new complexity. This indicator was not selected for detailed attention.

AIDS

The most dramatic new development affecting the health and survival of children is infection with the human immunosuppressive virus (HIV). First cases were recognized among children infected as a result of transmission by blood transfusions and the administration of blood products to treat hemophilia. By 1984, additional cases were recognized as a result of transplacental infection from mothers. Large numbers of children were diagnosed in population centers (New York City, Newark, and Miami) where adult cases of AIDS were most common. By early 1987, nearly 500 cases of AIDS in children had been diagnosed, and two to three times that number of children were presumed to be infected but not yet recognized. The Public Health Service estimates that by 1991 some 3,000 children will have contracted the disease and virtually all will die.[9]

In New York City, every 65th newborn was recently reported in newspaper accounts to have HIV antibodies. Some of these infants are infected; others only temporarily have their mothers' passively transmitted antibodies. Infected babies are born to mothers who themselves are infected through intravenous drug use or through heterosexual transmission from a partner who was bisexual or who injected drugs. Infection in children appears to be increasingly identified with prostitute mothers who are intravenous drug users.[9]

Many uncertainties surround these tragic events. To what extent will newly developed medications prolong life? Can vaccines be developed? What is the threat of widespread dissemination of infection among heterosexual couples? In the absence of answers to these questions, the best approaches require intensive research, diligent monitoring for infection, and widespread public education about the infection, its means of dissemination, and the protections that need to be taken against it. Although infants and young children have become the victims of the new epidemic, means of control need to focus on older populations.

Poverty

The poverty rate reached 22.2 children per 100 in 1983, the highest level since the mid-1960s. Between 1959 and 1969, the poverty rate for children was cut in half to a low of 13.8 in 1969,[3] but in the intervening years, children have replaced the elderly as the age group predominating among the nation's poor. Between 1983 and 1985, the overall poverty rate for children fell slightly, but the rate for Hispanic children increased.[12] A child's chances of being poor vary sharply by age, race, presence of the father, and marital status of the mother:

• Almost half of all black children and more than one-third of all Hispanic children are poor.

• Most children in female-headed households are poor. For children in black, female-headed families in which the mother is single, is under age 30, and did not complete high school, the poverty rate is 92.8%.

Careful documentation in recent years has established that children and pregnant women in poverty suffer excess mortality and morbidity by many measures;[13] they are underserved relative to their need;[7] and their health can be measurably improved by providing them with appropriate supports and services.[4] Data on the proportion of children living in poverty are readily available by census tract. This information has assumed growing importance as an indicator of areas where families and children require special attention.

Descriptions of the Indicators

The 12 measures described in this report include a number of traditional public health measures that are generally recognized by public health experts as reliable and important for program planning and for which data are systematically or universally collected in vital statistics. Examples are the infant mortality rate, rate of low birth weight babies, and rate of receipt of prenatal care. These traditional public health measures are included here in the belief that they need to be better understood by a broad lay and professional public, that scattered information about them should be brought together for convenient reference, and that they should not share in the mystification that surrounds so much material relating to the public's health and medical care.

The measures also include some that are well known by experts and have already had limited use in the formulation of child health policy, but that may become more influential if presented to the public and to policy makers with clearer definition and explanation of significance, or if data are collected more frequently or in a more representative or universal manner. Examples include elevated blood lead levels, population-based growth stunting, and severe iron deficiency anemia. This category of outcome indicators is included with the hope that they will be useful in raising consciousness about health issues that may be recognized by public health experts but require additional attention by the public and by health professionals who are schooled in case management, but not in the health needs of populations.

The indicators are organized according to their greatest age-specific relevance, although the separations are not absolute. For example, motor vehicle accident fatalities are a serious problem for all age groups, but the importance is especially great for teenagers and young adults. Similarly, non–motor vehicle accident fatalities have special significance as indicators of home safety for toddlers. Two of the indicators, child abuse and anemia, relate to all age groups. The 12 indicators are organized as follows:

Newborns and Infants

- Inadequate Prenatal Care
- Low Birth Weight Infants
- Infant Mortality Rate

Children

- Inadequate Immunization Status
- Population-Based Growth Stunting
- Elevated Blood Lead Levels
- Non–Motor Vehicle Accident Fatalities

Adolescents and Young Adults

- Births to School-Age Mothers
- Suicides
- Motor Vehicle Accident Fatalities

All Ages

- Iron Deficiency Anemia
- Child Abuse or Neglect

Each measure has been annotated with the following information:

- definition,

- exact indicator(s) to be used,
- health implications,
- policy implications,
- current status and trends,
- risk factors,
- 1990 U.S. Objectives,
- data sources (national, state, and local), and
- data needs and gaps.

The annotations are intended to be helpful to monitoring groups interested in identifying problem populations, linking changes in health status to changes in policies and programs, and advocating for policies and programs based on outcome data.

Citations of other sources of information are abundant but not exhaustive. If good review articles are available, they are cited in place of a complete listing of primary sources. Most of the references rely on authoritative refereed publications or on official reports from established agencies. In some instances, references to the publications of public interest groups are also included because the data are presented especially clearly or are more current than data available elsewhere.

Use of Indicators

As new interest focuses on the use of health outcome measures, consensus is emerging on the indicators that are most meaningful. The gradually increasing use of a defined and agreed-upon list of outcome indicators is fostering a new emphasis on predetermined objectives and accountability as a basis for decisions on resource allocation. Public bodies could be encouraged to apply outcome measures to defined populations, and providers for these populations might reasonably expect to be held accountable in those terms.

It is important to note that a movement toward basing child health policies on achieving specified health outcomes would allow states, localities, and provider systems the freedom to develop their own strategies to achieve these nationally agreed-upon outcomes in different ways. Differences in local needs, resources, and preferences could be expressed in different programs and strategies, while the responsibility to meet outcome standards protective of the public's interest would be preserved.

In the long run, health outcome indicators can become a means of educating the public and policy makers regarding some of the important facts about child health and child health policy that seem to have been neglected and overlooked in the recent past. A clear focus on outcomes can promote greater recognition and acceptance of a number of important concepts, including the following:

- Child health needs and ways of meeting these needs are not exclusively medical issues. Child health must be viewed in a complex social and environmental context, and effective approaches to unmet child health problems use currently available scientific knowledge, cut across professional disciplines and helping systems, and require attention to issues in the realms of medicine and health, mental health, education, social services, corrections, employment, income distribution, housing, and day care.
- Wide disparities in health status among various population groups can be reduced by improving the nature of, quality of, availability of, and access to health and health-related services.
- Currently available opportunities for preventing disease, disability, and unnecessary suffering require a reorienting of economic incentives, of many aspects of the training of health professionals, and of the organization and delivery of many health and health-related services. Also required is a better way of bringing the findings of biomedical and behavioral sciences to bear on the practice of medicine and public health. The currently unrealized opportunities for preventive intervention are particularly great during pregnancy, early childhood, and adolescence.

Ultimately, the use of child health outcome indicators is aimed at the development of just and effective policies and programs that promote the health and well-being of children. Although this goal cannot be achieved solely on the basis of the use of health outcome measures, the use of such measures is an important starting point, that deserves the attention of monitoring and advocacy groups, government data collectors, researchers, policy makers, and the general public.

Disaggregation of Data and Hazards of Interpretation

Among the 1990 Objectives for the Nation, those for maternal and child health are unique in specifying objectives for racial, socioeconomic, and geographic subgroups. At the hearings held to revise objectives for the year 2000, testimony emphasized that a similar approach should be taken throughout the new objectives lest aggregate data mask the persistence of neglect and serious problems among vulnerable populations.

Throughout the analysis of the 12 indicators in this report, data are disaggregated, often by race. This practice is well intentioned, and its potential advantages are obvious for targeting resources and interventions toward populations most in need. But there are hazards of interpretation.

In the United States, scant data are available on socioeconomic levels, but vital statistics are full of information on race, age, and marital status. We tend to report data that are available and to interpret them by relying on known associations. Unless great care is exercised, discriminatory stereotypes can be perpetuated. Dysfunctional families occur among all races and all socioeconomic levels. If we had readily accessible measures of family dysfunction, we would understand better the dynamics of such outcomes as child abuse, teenage pregnancy, low birth weight, and high infant mortality.[10] Lacking that information, we risk burdening minorities, teenagers, and unmarried mothers with stereotypes they do not deserve. We must strive harder to identify the influences that contribute to the poor health outcomes associated with these subgroups and try even harder to understand the interventions and supports that can help them realize the many assets of individuality that are cherished by each of us.

References

1. American Public Health Association. Model standards: a guide for community preventive health services. 2nd ed. Washington, DC: APHA, 1985.

2. Centers for Disease Control. Model standards for community preventive health services. DHEW Pub. No. 1980–640–185/4430. Washington, DC: CDC, 1979.

3. Congressional Research Service. Children in poverty. Committee of Ways and Means, U.S. House of Representatives, U.S. Congress. Washington, DC: CRS, 1985.

4. Egbuonu L, Starfield B. Child health and social status. Pediatrics 1982;69:550–6.

5. Massell BF, Chute C, Walker A, Kurland G. Penicillin and the marked decrease in morbidity and mortality from rheumatic fever in the US. N Engl J Med 1988;318(5):280–6.

6. McGinnis J. Setting nationwide objectives in disease prevention and health promotion: the United States experience. In: Holland WW, Detels RT, Knox G, eds. Oxford textbook of public health; vol 3, Investigation methods in public health. Oxford, England: Oxford University Press, 1985:385–401.

7. Newacheck P. Access to ambulatory care services for economically disadvantaged children. Pediatrics 1986;78:813–9.

8. Public Health Service. Promoting health/preventing disease: objectives for the nation. DHHS Pub. No. (OM)81–0007. Washington, DC: PHS, 1980.

9. Public Health Service. Report of the Surgeon General's Workshop in Children with HIV infection and their families. U.S. Department of Health and Human Services. Washington, DC: PHS, 1987.

10. Reeb K, Graham A, Zyzanski S, Gayck. Predicting low birthweight and complicated labor in urban black women: a biophysical perspective. Soc Sci Med 1987;25(12):1321–7.

11. Rutstein D, Berenberg W, Chalmers T, Childs C, Fishman A, Perrin E. Measuring the quality of medical care. N Engl J Med 1976;294:582–8.

12. Select Committee on Children, Youth, and Families. US children and their families: current conditions and recent trends, 1987. U.S. House of Representatives, U.S. Congress. Washington, DC: GPO, 1987.

13. Starfield B. Child health and socioeconomic status. Amer J Public Health 1982;72:532–3.

14. Zill N, Petersen J, Moore K. Improving national statistics on children, youth, and families. Washington, DC: Child Trends, 1984.

CHAPTER 2

Indicators of Special Importance to Newborns and Infants

Inadequate Prenatal Care

Definition

Prenatal care is defined as pregnancy-related health care services provided to a woman between conception and delivery. These services are aimed at preventing poor outcomes for both mother and baby. Although prenatal care varies with the setting, provider, and patient, it should include the following: regular assessments and care of the physical health of the mother and fetus, including genetic screening for selected populations; education on nutrition, exercise, health habits, birth preparation, and baby care; special benefits as needed, such as supplemental foods; a psychosocial component aimed at assuring adequate support systems for the mother and family; and planning for labor, delivery, and postnatal care, including family planning. The recommended schedule of care developed by the American College of Obstetrics and Gynecology is a minimum of one health care visit in the first 13 weeks, followed by one visit per month until the 28th week, a visit every two weeks until the 36th week of pregnancy, and weekly visits thereafter. This schedule has come under question for providing insufficient opportunity for counseling early in pregnancy.

Indicator

- The proportion of births to mothers who received delayed prenatal care (starting in the third trimester) or no prenatal care at all.

Significance

Although prenatal care is a process indicator, its use is appropriate because of its strong association with pregnancy outcome, especially among poor and minority populations. The prenatal care that women receive is the second most important determinant of birth outcome,[14] after socioeconomic status.

The rate of participation in prenatal care should be a particularly useful measure when data on related outcomes (infant mortality and low birth weight) are difficult to obtain or of questionable significance, as with data on small populations or for short time spans. In general, data on prenatal care reflect changes in policy and programs sooner than data on low birth weight or infant mortality.

Health Implications

Pregnant women who receive inadequate prenatal care are at increased risk of bearing infants who are low birth weight, are stillborn, or die within the first year of life. Infants born with low birth weight or needing neonatal intensive care do better if their mothers received prenatal services than if their mothers received no care prior to delivery.[15, 28]

Inadequate prenatal care is also linked to specific diseases or disorders of newborns that could have been diagnosed and treated under proper supervision of a trained health care provider—for example, congenital syphilis or newborn hemolytic anemia resulting from a blood incompatibility between the mother and the fetus.

Comprehensive prenatal care incorporates many interventions designed to improve pregnancy outcome by encouraging health-promoting behavior. For example, pregnant smokers who participate in smoking reduction programs have been found to increase the average weight of their babies. Nutrition supplementation, counseling, and home visiting also have been associated with increased birth weight. Yet another intervention presumed to favor improved health for infant and mother is the reduction of both physical and emotional stress during pregnancy. Although the research basis for this presumption is less than firm, most European countries forbid strenuous or night work for pregnant women. In this country, demonstration projects featuring stress reduction have yielded promising results.[4, 10, 17, 29]

Policy and Program Implications

The proportion of women failing to receive adequate prenatal care is an important indicator of a society's commitment to provide the most basic preventive services aimed at improving pregnancy outcome and maintaining women's health. A higher than average proportion of women receiving inadequate prenatal care among certain population groups, especially those of low socioeconomic or educational status, reflects deficiencies in public programs intended to assure acceptable and equitable access to essential health services. In addition, because very young, unmarried, poor and minority women are already at increased risk of poor pregnancy outcome, if a higher than average proportion of these women receive inadequate prenatal care, a misallocation of health resources is implied, with people who are most needy receiving the least adequate care.

Research suggests that, although the association between receipt of prenatal care and improved pregnancy outcome holds for all sociodemographic groups, the relative strength of this association varies with race, education, and income. These differences may be obscured, however, if a single estimate of effect is calculated for the aggregate population. The impact of prenatal care on pregnancy outcome appears to be most substantial for black women in general and for both black and white women who are poor (as measured by delivery on general versus private hospital services), poorly educated, or both.[7] An analysis of the increase in risk attributable to inadequate prenatal care suggests that the greatest improvement in pregnancy outcome (as measured by low birth weight) can be expected if programs are targeted to the most socially disadvantaged groups.[9]

Cost-Effectiveness of Prenatal Care

Receipt of adequate prenatal care can help contain health care costs by preventing conditions that require expensive treatment. It is estimated that by providing prenatal and postpartum preventive health care to all low-income women, the federal government could save more than $360 million per year in costs for neonatal intensive care and rehospitalization of low birth weight infants.[3] By reducing the risk of chronic handicapping conditions, prenatal care can also reduce the incalculable costs for future medical care, special schooling, and social services.

The Institute of Medicine's Committee to Study the Prevention of Low Birthweight has urged adoption of a national program to assure equitable access to comprehensive prenatal care for all pregnant women. It is estimated that every dollar invested in such a program would save $3.38 in subsequent expenditures for the care of low birth weight babies.[13]

The American Academy of Pediatrics reports that cost-benefit analyses show between $2 and $10 saved for every dollar spent on prenatal care.[1]

Status and Trends

National

• In 1985, 5.6% of live births in the United States (approximately 1 out of 18) were to women who received late or no prenatal care. This was the third consecutive year for which the proportion of babies born to women receiving late or no prenatal care remained constant.[20]

• Between 1984 and 1985, the proportion of babies born to women receiving late or no prenatal care increased among blacks (from 9.6% to 10.3%) and remained constant for whites (4.7%).[12, 20]

• Between 1970 and 1979, the United States witnessed a steady decrease in the percentage of all women receiving late or no prenatal care, with a greater decline among blacks than among whites (declines of 35% for all races, 46% for blacks, and 31% for whites). In the 1980s, these favorable trends have been reversed. From 1980 to 1985, the receipt of late or no prenatal care increased 10% for all races, 9% for whites, and 17% for blacks.[12, 20]

• Black women are more than twice as likely as white women to receive late or no prenatal care. In 1985, 10.3% of births to blacks, as compared with 4.7% of births to whites, were to women receiving third-trimester care or no care at all.[20]

• Hispanic women in the United States are at even greater risk than blacks of receiving inadequate care. In 1985, 12.4% of Hispanic-origin mothers did not begin prenatal care until the third trimester of pregnancy or received no prenatal care at all.[33]

• Of all age groups, teens are most likely to delay prenatal care or receive no care at all. In 1985, 20.5% of mothers under age 15 and 12.0% of mothers aged 15 through 19 received late or no prenatal care.[20]

• Poor women in the United States are three times more likely than women who are not poor to receive late or no prenatal care.[30]

• Overall, unmarried women in the United States are four times as likely as married women to delay prenatal care or receive no care at all.[30]

• Women without health insurance are at greatly increased risk of receiving delayed or no prenatal care. Among women who arrive at the hospital for delivery without insurance, the proportion who have received no prenatal care is four times the national average. The Alan Guttmacher Institute reports that 14.6 million women in their childbearing years have no insurance coverage (either public or private) for maternity care. Of these, more than half a million give birth each year, accounting for 15% of births in the United States.[6]

• According to the Institute of Medicine, there are six major barriers to receipt of timely prenatal care for American women: financial constraints; limited availability of maternity care providers, especially for socially disadvantaged women; insufficient prenatal services, especially at sites used by high-risk women; experiences, attitudes, and beliefs that discourage women from seeking prenatal care; inadequate transportation and child care services; and inadequate recruitment of hard-to-reach populations.[13]

• Government Accounting Office (GAO) researchers studying barriers to prenatal care in 8 states and 32 communities found that most women face multiple barriers, with three predominating in virtually every community: "lack of money to pay for care, lack of transportation to get to the provider of care and lack of awareness of the pregnancy."[8]

• GAO analysts report that 63% of women who receive Medicaid encounter problems establishing eligibility during their pregnancies. GAO concludes that an important barrier to early care could be removed if women could receive services while waiting for Medicaid to establish their eligibility (presumptive eligibility). GAO analysts further conclude that states with limited resources might be most successful in expanding access to care if they both establish presumptive eligibility and expand eligibility to cover pregnant women living up to 100% of the poverty level.[8]

• Although information is readily available on the proportion of women receiving prenatal care and on the timing of this care, very little is known about the current components of prenatal care, their efficacy and safety, and how they should be combined to meet the needs of particular populations.[13] Such information is needed to establish both optimal services and insurance coverage for these services.[6]

State and Local

• Between 1984 and 1985, 32 states experienced increases in the percentage of women receiving late or no prenatal care, and 29 experienced declines in the percentage of women receiving early (first-trimester) care.[11]

• In 1985, New Mexico had the largest percentage of women receiving late or no prenatal care (13.4%) and Iowa had the smallest percentage (2.1%).[11]

• A Lea County, New Mexico, study of women receiving no prenatal care found that 77% stated they had not received prenatal care because they could not afford it.[2]

• Researchers from the University of California in San Diego report that the cost of providing comprehensive prenatal care to predominantly Hispanic women and their infants is considerably less than the cost of providing little or no prenatal care to the same population. Perinatal costs per mother-infant pair were $2974 for those enrolled in a comprehensive perinatal program and $5168 for those who received three or fewer prenatal visits.[18]

• The Missouri Department of Health Statistics reports that pregnant women participating in the Special Supplemental Food Program for Women, Infants, and Children (WIC) save the state an average of $100 each in Medicaid costs. The state found WIC participation to be associated with reductions in low birth weight and in admission to neonatal intensive care.[28]

• In Washington State, researchers have linked increases in receipt of late or no prenatal care to the economic recession of the early 1980s. Between 1980 and 1982, the proportion of births to women receiving delayed or no care increased 32% in low-income areas and 44% in higher income areas of the state.[5]

Risk Factors

Women at increased risk of receiving late or no prenatal care include nonwhite women, women who are poor or poorly educated, teenagers and women over age 45, women with three or more previous pregnancies, and unmarried women.

U.S. Objective for Prenatal Care

In 1980 the U.S. Department of Health and Human Services (HHS) established the following objective for receipt of prenatal care:

- By 1990, the proportion of women in any county or racial or ethnic group (white, black, Hispanic, or American Indian) who obtained no prenatal care during the first trimester of pregnancy should not exceed 10%.[26] (In 1980, 20.7% of white mothers, 37.3% of black mothers, 39.8% of Hispanic mothers, and 41.3% of American Indian mothers received no prenatal care during the first trimester.[19, 32])

In a 1985 report to Congress, the Department of Health and Human Services projected that

> The national objective for early participation in prenatal care will not be attained by either white or black mothers in 1990. State-by-state projections indicate that even among whites, only Maine and New Hampshire will meet the national objective.[16]

Data Sources

State and Local

The most timely state and local data are available from each state's bureau of vital statistics (usually within the state health department), which is responsible for collecting birth certificate data that will eventually be sent to the National Center for Health Statistics (NCHS). Most states publish birth data annually, including information on receipt of prenatal care. All states now link birth and death certificates, either by computer or manually. Some use the linked birth-death records to tabulate infant deaths by receipt of prenatal care. Some states provide birth statistics by census tract. These data can be related to data on socioeconomic status, also available by census tract.

In large cities. the city or county health department (vital statistics registrar) may publish data on receipt of prenatal care. Smaller cities tend to rely on state publication of data.

The NCHS publication *Advance Report of Final Natality Statistics,*[20] part of the Monthly Vital Statistics Report series, provides state data on live births by month in pregnancy that prenatal care was begun, number of prenatal visits, and race of child.

The Children's Defense Fund, Washington, DC, provides a wealth of state and local data on receipt of prenatal care in its annual publication *The Health of America's Children: Maternal and Child Health Data Book.*[11] The data book includes a ranking of states by mother's entry into prenatal care, a similar ranking for teen mothers, a year-by-year listing for each state showing the percentage of births to mothers receiving early prenatal care and the percentage to mothers receiving late or no prenatal care, and an analysis of each state's progress toward meeting the Surgeon General's 1990 Objectives for the Nation.

National

National data on prenatal care are available from the NCHS Vital Statistics Registration System (VSRS), which receives continuous data from states based on information required on birth certificates. Since 1968, the standardized birth certificate adopted by most states has included two questions pertaining to prenatal care: month of pregnancy in which prenatal care began and total number of visits. The most complete information is reported in the annual NCHS publication *Vital Statistics of the United States, Vol. 1, Natality,*[21] which provides data on receipt of prenatal care tabulated by race, birth weight, and birth order of infant, and by education and marital status of mother. There is a three- to four-year lag between the end of a calendar year and publication of data for that year. However, all of the data are available once final natality statistics are reported in the NCHS Monthly Vital Statistics Report series (discussed next).

A more timely, but less complete source of national data is the NCHS *Advance Report of Final Natality Statistics,*[20] which is part of the Monthly Vital Statistics Report series and presents data on live births by month of pregnancy in which prenatal care began and total number of prenatal visits tabulated by race and age of mother. The *Advance Report* is available approximately 1.5 to 2 years after the end of a calendar year.

The Children's Defense Fund publication *The Health of America's Children: Maternal and Child Health Data Book*[11] includes discussion of national progress in meeting the Surgeon General's 1990 Objectives for prenatal care; data on prenatal care and birth outcome, by age; and a year-by-year listing by race of the percentage of births to women receiving early prenatal care and to women receiving late or no prenatal care (starting with 1969 data).

The National Natality Surveys (NNS), conducted by NCHS in 1963–69, 1972, and 1980, provide periodic data on receipt of prenatal care by characteristics beyond those covered on birth certificates, such as mother's occupation and work history during pregnancy, father's occupation, source of medical care for mother and infant, and family income. Data from the NNS are periodically available in a variety of publications, including reports in the Vital and Health Statistics series and supplements to the Monthly Vital Statistics Report series. Data from the 1980 NNS have been analyzed in a broad range of papers and publications, most of which are available from the Natality Branch of NCHS.[24] Public-use data tapes of the follow-back surveys are available from the National Technical Information Service (NTIS). Data collection for the next NNS, called the National Maternal and Infant Health Survey, began in the fall of 1988 and will continue through 1990. The survey will include data on barriers to and facilitators of prenatal care; exercise and bed rest during pregnancy; use and evaluation of public programs, such as WIC and Medicaid; and maternal and infant rehospitalization after delivery.[25]

Both the Centers for Disease Control (CDC) and NCHS have recently initiated projects that evaluate linked birth-death certificate data, thus helping to clarify the relationship between receipt of prenatal care and infant mortality. The CDC's National Infant Mortality Surveillance Project (NIMS) compiled the states' linked birth-death records to analyze data for the 1980 birth cohort. Findings have been reported in a special section of *Public Health Reports*.[27] Additional state-specific data from NIMS will be published and will be available on public-use data tapes in the future. The Linked Birth and Infant Death Record Project of NCHS is currently funded to link and analyze birth-death certificate data from the 1983–86 birth cohorts. It is anticipated that, starting with the 1987 cohort, this much-needed national data base will become part of routine data collection and reporting by NCHS. Public-use data tapes for the 1983 birth cohort should be available in March 1989. Tapes and publications for subsequent birth cohorts will be available in the future.

Useful reviews of currently available data are found in *Healthy Children. Investing in the Future*[23] and in *Disease Prevention/Health Promotion: The Facts.*[22]

Data Needs

State and Local

In response to an apparent reduction in the timely provision of prenatal care and a general slowing of the decline in the infant mortality rate, the Public Health Service has assembled a cadre of health professionals to provide expert assistance to states to conduct infant mortality reviews and investigations of conditions associated with high or changing infant mortality. The approach is designed to assist state health departments in gaining a better understanding of the nature of local difficulties in reducing infant mortality. In addition, it assists in gathering precise information concerning local maternal and infant health care systems and opportunities for improvement.

National

There are several problems with the national data system regarding prenatal care. One gap has been the absence of ongoing national data linking receipt of care to infant mortality. At long last, it appears that this gap will be filled if, as anticipated, the Linked Birth and Infant Death Record Project of NCHS becomes part of routine data collection and reporting of the Vital Statistics Registration System.

A second shortcoming of the current national data system is the considerable time lag between the end of a calendar year and publication of final national data for that year. There is a lag of approximately one to four years before publication of final VSRS data on receipt of prenatal care. In addition, it is projected that national linked birth-death certificate data for any given birth cohort may not be available until approximately four years after the year of birth. This relatively long lag makes it difficult to use timely national prenatal care data in evaluating, planning, and implementing public policies.

National prenatal care data by income (or class, as the British use) are very limited. Although the NNS does provide periodic data by income, the VSRS does not collect this information. As a result, surrogate measures such as race or mother's education are often used, making it more difficult to distinguish to what extent low birth weight is associated with poverty as distinct from other factors.

Although the NNS collects information from married mothers on participation in public programs, there is no national data base that systematically and continuously links prenatal care data to participation in public programs such as WIC, Medicaid, and Aid to Families with Dependent Children (AFDC). This information, if linked with data on income or class, would be particularly useful in evaluating the impact of public policies and programs.

National data collected by ethnicity are not complete. Although the VSRS collects prenatal care data by ethnicity, reporting by states is uneven. National data on receipt of prenatal care by women of Hispanic origin were first available for the 1978 birth cohort, based on reporting from 17 states. The 1985 data on Hispanics are based on reporting from 23 states and the District of Columbia.[33] Data on prenatal care of women of Asian origin (Chinese, Filipino, Japanese, Hawaiian, and other) were first published by NCHS in 1984.[31]

References

1. American Academy of Pediatrics. Child health financing report. Evanston, IL: AAP, 1984.

2. Berger L. Public/private cooperation in rural maternal child health efforts: the Lea County Perinatal Program. Texas Medicine 1984;80(Sep):54–7.

3. Blackwell A, Salisbury L, Arriola A. An administrative petition to the United States Department of Health and Human Services. San Francisco: Public Advocates, 1983.

4. Buescher P. Source of prenatal care and infant birthweight: the case of a North Carolina county. State Center for Health Statistics Studies, No. 39. Raleigh, NC: North Carolina Department of Human Resources, 1986.

5. Fisher E, LoGerfo J, Daling J. Prenatal care and pregnancy outcomes during the recession: the Washington State experience. Am J Public Health 1985;75(8):866–9.

6. Gold R, Kenney A, Singh S. Blessed events and the bottom line: financing maternity care in the United States. New York: Alan Guttmacher Institute, 1987.

7. Gortmaker S. The effect of prenatal care upon the health of the newborn. Am J Public Health 1979;69(7):653–60.

8. Government Accounting Office. Prenatal care: Medicaid recipients and uninsured women obtain insufficient care. Report to the U.S. House of Representatives. GAO Pub. No. (GAO/HRD) 87–137. Washington, DC: GAO, 1987.

9. Greenberg R. The impact of prenatal care in different social groups. Am J Obstet Gynecol 1983;145(7):797–801.

10. Hobel C. A randomized assessment of low birthweight prevention interventions. Perspective on Prevention 1988;2(3):19–23.

11. Hughes D, Johnson K, Rosenbaum S, Butler E, Simons J. The health of America's children: maternal and child health data book. Washington, DC: Children's Defense Fund, 1988.

12. Hughes D, Johnson K, Rosenbaum S, Simons J, Butler E. The health of America's children: maternal and child health data book. Washington, DC: Children's Defense Fund, 1987.

13. Institute of Medicine. Preventing low birthweight. Washington, DC: National Academy Press, 1985.

14. Kessner D. Contrasts in health status. Vol 1, Infant death: an analysis by maternal risk and health care. Washington, DC: Institute of Medicine, National Academy of Sciences, 1973.

15. Leveno K, Cunningham F, Roark M, Nelson S, Williams M. Prenatal care and the low-birth weight infant. Obstet Gynecol 1985;66(Nov):1439–44.

16. Mason J. Report to the Subcommittee on Oversight and Investigation of the Committee on Energy and Commerce, U.S. House of Representatives, 3 Apr. Washington, DC: U.S. Department of Health and Human Services, 1985.

17. Miller C. Maternal and infant survival. Washington, DC: National Center for Clinical Infant Programs, 1987.

18. Moore T, Origel W, Key T, Resnik R. The perinatal and economic impact of prenatal care in a low-socioeconomic population. Am J Obstet Gynecol 1986;154(Jan):29–33.

19. National Center for Health Statistics. Health—United States, 1983. DHHS Pub. No. (PHS)84–1232. Washington, DC: NCHS, 1983.

20. National Center for Health Statistics. Advance report of final natality statistics, 1985. Monthly Vital Statistics Report 36(4). Supplement. DHHS Pub. No. (PHS)87–1120. Washington, DC: NCHS, 1987.

21. National Center for Health Statistics. Vital statistics of the United States, 1985. Vol. 1, Natality. DHHS Pub. No. (PHS) 87–1113. Washington, DC: NCHS, 1987.

22. Office of Disease Prevention and Health Promotion. Disease prevention health promotion: the facts. U.S. Public Health Service. Department of Health and Human Services Bulletin. Palo Alto, CA: ODPHP, 1988.

23. Office of Technology Assessment. Healthy children, investing in the future. Congress of the United States. Washington, DC: OTA, 1987.

24. Placek P. One hundred and twenty-five (125) reports, papers, and publications using the 1980 Natality Survey and the 1980 National Fetal Mortality Survey. Washington, DC: National Center for Health Statistics, 1987.

25. Placek P. 1988 National Maternal and Infant Health Survey. Washington, DC: National Center for Health Statistics, 1988.

26. Public Health Service. Promoting health preventing disease: objectives for the nation. DHHS Pub. No. (OM)81–0007. Washington, DC: PHS, 1980.

27. Public Health Service. Special section—national surveillance of infant mortality. Public Health Reports 1987;102(Mar–Apr):126–216.

28. Schramm W. WIC prenatal participation and its relationship to newborn Medicaid costs in Missouri: a cost/benefit analysis. Am J Public Health 1985;75(8):851–7.

29. Sexton M, Hebel J. A clinical trial of change in maternal smoking and its effect on birth weight. JAMA 1984;251(7):911–5.

30. Singh S, Torres A, Forrest J. The need for prenatal care in the United States: evidence from the 1980 National Natality Survey. Fam Plann Perspect 1985;17(3):118–24.

31. Taffel S. Characteristics of Asian births: United States, 1980. Monthly Vital Statistics Report 32(10). Supplement. DHHS Publ. No. (PHS)84–1120. Washington, DC: National Center for Health Statistics, 1984.

32. Ventura S. Births of Hispanic parentage, 1980. Monthly Vital Statistics Report 32(6). Supplement. DHHS Pub. No. (PHS)83–1120. Washington, DC: National Center for Health Statistics, 1983.

33. Ventura S. Births of Hispanic parentage, 1985. Monthly Vital Statistics Report 36(11). Supplement. DHHS Pub. No. (PHS)88-1120. Washington, DC: National Center for Health Statistics, 1988.

Low Birth Weight Infants

Definition

Low birth weight (LBW) infants are infants weighing less than 2500 g (5.5 lb) at birth. They fall into two categories: those who are small because they are born prematurely (fewer than 37 weeks of gestation completed) and those who are full-term babies, but are small for their gestational age (intrauterine growth retardation).

Indicator

- The number of infants weighing less than 2500 g (5.5 lb) at birth per 100 live births (LBW rate).

Significance

Health Implications

LBW infants are at increased risk of suffering severe physical and developmental complications and death. In the United States, these infants account for nearly two-thirds of all deaths under 28 days of age (neonatal deaths) and 60% of all infant deaths in the first year of life.[12, 28] Compared with other infants, LBW babies are almost 40 times more likely to die in the first month of life and are 5 times more likely to die between one month and one year of age (postneonatal death).[4]

Despite reductions over the past 20 years in the rate of severely handicapping conditions associated with LBW, the LBW infants who survive are still at increased risk of mental retardation, birth defects, growth and developmental problems, visual and hearing defects, delayed speech, autism, cerebral palsy, epilepsy, learning difficulties, chronic lung problems, and abuse and neglect. Risks are greatly increased for infants born weighing less than 1500 g and for those requiring artificial ventilation.[4, 11, 16, 18, 19, 20, 28, 39]. Pregnant women who were themselves LBW babies are at increased risk of poor pregnancy outcome.[10]

Policy and Program Implications

The LBW rate is an important indicator of the health and welfare of a population. Higher LBW rates among subpopulations of our society reflect disparities in socioeconomic and educational status, access to early and continuous maternity care, and adequate prenatal nutrition. In addition, LBW reflects maternal health behaviors such as smoking and alcohol consumption.

Costs of Low Birth Weight

The Institute of Medicine (IOM) estimates that $1.5 billion is spent annually in the United States to provide neonatal intensive care services, and the "vast majority of [this money] is spent for underweight infants."[4]

Status and Trends

National

• In 1985, 6.8% of all infants born in the United States—253,554 babies—were classified as low birth weight. This was the first increase in the national LBW rate in 20 years. The rate for 1984 was 6.7%. The proportion of low weight births remained constant in 1985 for both blacks (12.4%) and whites (5.6%). [15, 34]

• Internationally, the United States ranks 17th among selected countries in the percentage of babies born at low birth weight. Norway, Sweden, the Netherlands, Finland, Ireland, Switzerland, France, Japan, the Federal Republic of Germany, Belgium, Austria, Greece, Canada, Denmark, the German Democratic Republic, and Italy all have a lower incidence of low birth weight than the United States.[14]

• The LBW rate in the United States in 1985 (6.8%) was identical to the rate in 1980 and was only slightly lower than the rate of 7.4% in 1975.[15] Almost all (86%) of the decline in the LBW rate in the past decade took place between 1975 and 1980, and virtually all of this decline was among moderately LBW infants (1500–2499 g). Between 1975 and 1985, the proportion of very LBW infants (less than 1500 g) increased for all races.[32, 34, 35]

• Black infants are three times as likely as white infants to be very low birth weight and more than twice as likely to be moderately low birth weight. This disparity between the races is associated both with a greater frequency of preterm births among black infants and with a higher frequency of LBW among term and postterm black infants.[21, 44]

• Over the past 30 years, the gap between white and nonwhite LBW rates has increased. This widening gap reflects two distinct trends: First, from 1950 through the mid-1960s, the LBW rate for nonwhites rose sharply, while the rate for whites rose only slightly. (Recent analysis suggests that the rise in LBW among nonwhites may reflect better reporting of LBW due to a major increase in hospital-based births for the nonwhite population during these years.) Second, from the mid-1960s to the present, the general decline in LBW was slower for nonwhites than for whites. The ratios of nonwhite to white LBW for the years 1950, 1965, and 1985 were, respectively, 1.52, 1.93, and 1.98.[7, 34, 44]

• Babies who are born prematurely are at greatly increased risk of being low birth weight: 39.4% of preterm infants, compared with 3.0% of term infants, are born low birth weight. Between 1984 and 1985, the proportion of all U.S. infants born preterm increased from 9.4% to 9.8%. This increase is consistent with the trend in recent years for all races, for blacks, and for whites. Between 1980 and 1985, the proportion of preterm infants increased among whites from 7.9% to 8.2% and among blacks from 16.8% to 17.5%, thus maintaining the racial gap.[34]

• Recent research highlights the need to better understand racial disparities in low birth weight. Although it is clear that blacks and other minorities are more likely than white to be characterized as high risk in terms of factors such as maternal age, parity, marital status, and educational level, the extent to which racial disparities persist once these and other known risk factors are controlled remains a topic of debate. Most researchers agree that although further research into the causes of LBW may be needed, we know enough now about some interventions that do work to begin targeting resources and tailoring programs to reach blacks and other minorities at greatest risk.[1, 2, 21, 25, 40]

• The weight of informed opinion holds that the presence of the sickle cell trait (heterozygosity) does not increase a pregnant woman's risk of having an LBW infant. However, nearly all writers agree that urinary tract infections during pregnancy are greatly increased among women with the sickle cell trait.[29] This finding is noteworthy in view of reports that high rates of urinary tract infections persist as a risk factor for low birth weight, even as all other known variables are corrected.[30]

• The proportion of LBW infants born to Mexican and Central and South American women in the United States compares favorably with the proportion of LBW infants born to white non-Hispanic women. In 1984, the proportion of LBW infants was 5.7% among Mexicans, 5.8% for Central and South Americans, 5.5% among Cubans, and 5.5% among other white non-Hispanics. The rate for Puerto Rican babies, however, was 8.9%. Further data indicate that among Hispanic women giving birth in the Unites States, those who are foreign-born are less likely than those who are U.S.-

born to bear LBW infants. The relatively small proportion of low weight births among most Hispanic groups in the United States is of particular interest because, relative to white non-Hispanic women, Hispanic women have lower levels of maternal education, higher levels of poverty, and lower participation in prenatal care, all characteristics generally associated with increased risk of low birth weight. Factors that may help explain the relatively few low weight births among Hispanics include both a reduced incidence of smoking and an increased emphasis on good prenatal nutrition among Hispanics as compared with non-Hispanics.[48, 50]

• Teenagers are much more likely to give birth to LBW infants than are mothers in their 20s, and the risks are greatest among the youngest teenagers. In 1985, 12.9% of mothers under age 15, compared with 5.9% of mothers ages 25 through 29, gave birth to LBW infants. Among mothers ages 15 through 19, the LBW rate was 9.3%.[34] Although low birth weight is certainly a serious problem among infants born to teenaged mothers, the relative contribution of teenage childbearing to the overall problem of low birth weight may have been overstated in recent years. In 1983, for example, infants of teenaged mothers accounted for 8% of low weight births among whites and only 3% among blacks.[21]

• Children born into poverty are at increased risk of being low birth weight. The National Center for Health Statistics (NCHS) reports that even in areas where voluntary (private) and public hospitals have the same racial mix, the incidence of LBW babies runs 40% to 50% higher in public hospitals.[33]

• Infants whose mothers received no prenatal care are three times more likely to be low birth weight than are infants whose mothers started care in the first three months of pregnancy. Based on 1981 data, the Institute of Medicine reports that if all women in the United States received prenatal care starting in the first three months of pregnancy, LBW could be reduced by 15% among whites and by 12% among blacks.[4]

• Women who smoke during pregnancy are more likely to bear LBW infants than are nonsmokers. An analysis of data from the 1980 NNS indicates that among married white non-Hispanic women 20 through 34 years old, the odds of bearing a LBW baby increase 26% for every five cigarettes smoked per day. Further, it is estimated that among this study population the incidence of LBW could be dramatically reduced if women would stop smoking during pregnancy, with the greatest declines among the least educated (who are most likely to smoke). Estimated reductions in low birth weight are 35% for women with less than 12 years of education, 20% for women with 12 years, and 11% for women with more than 12 years.[22]

- Participation in the federally funded WIC program (Special Supplemental Food Program for Women, Infants, and Children) is associated with decreases in low birth weight. Several studies indicate that the impact of the program is greater for blacks than for whites. Programs such as WIC might well have a greater overall impact on low birth weight in the United States if all eligible women could participate. It is estimated that in 1984 only 40% of eligible women were served by the program nationwide. [8, 23, 43, 47]

- The Institute of Medicine calculates that the United States could save from $12 to $29 million annually in medical services to LBW infants by providing early prenatal care (starting in the first three months of pregnancy) to a target population of virtually all poor and poorly educated pregnant women (aged 15–39, with less than 12 years of education, and receiving public assistance). This is considered a conservative estimate because it covers only the first year of medical expenses and does not include long-term costs of caring for handicapping conditions related to low birth weight. The IOM Committee to Study the Prevention of Low Birthweight concludes that the relationship between prenatal care and low birth weight is "strong enough to support a broad, national commitment to ensuring that all pregnant women in the United States, especially those at medical or socioeconomic risk, receive high quality prenatal care."[17]

State and Local

- Between 1984 and 1985, the LBW rate for whites increased in 21 states and the District of Columbia. The LBW rate for blacks increased in 18 states and the District of Columbia (data for blacks based on the 35 jurisdictions with at least 1,000 black births in 1985).[34]

- The highest proportion of low weight births in 1985 occurred predominantly in the South: the District of Columbia (13.3%), Mississippi (8.8%), Louisiana (8.7%), South Carolina (8.6%), Georgia (8.1%), Alabama (8.0%), Arkansas (8.0%), North Carolina (7.9%), Tennessee (7.9%), and Colorado (7.7%). The high rates of LBW in the South can in part be attributed to the relatively large black population in the region. But blacks in the South do not necessarily fare worse than in the rest of the nation. In 1985, the highest proportion of LBW among blacks occurred in the District of Columbia (15.3%), Michigan (13.6%), Connecticut (13.5%), Illinois (13.5%), Pennsylvania (13.4%), Colorado

(13.1%), Louisiana (13.1%), South Carolina (13.0%), Delaware (12.9%), Missouri (12.9%), and Tennessee (12.9%).[14] Only half of these are Southern.

• A study of the 85 poorest rural counties in the United States revealed significantly higher LBW rates in these areas than in the rest of the nation— 8.7% compared with 6.8% in 1983. This gap between poor rural and all other U.S. counties grew by 34% between 1980 and 1983.[41]

• In 1985, among U.S. cities with populations greater than 500,000, the District of Columbia had the greatest proportion of low weight births (13.3%), followed by Detroit (12.4%), Baltimore (12.0%), New Orleans (11.9%), and Memphis (10.5%).[14]

• Researchers in Alameda County, CA, found that women who reported financial problems during their pregnancies experienced nearly a sixfold increase in the risk of bearing a LBW infant.[3]

• In Missouri, WIC participation was associated with a 16% decrease in the proportion of infants who are low birth weight (22% decrease for blacks and 10% decrease for whites) and a 27% decrease in the proportion of very low birth weight infants.[43]

• In Guilford County, NC, poor women receiving comprehensive prenatal care from the County Health Department were far less likely to bear LBW infants than were poor women whose prenatal care was provided by private physicians and financed through Medicaid. Even after diverse risk factors were statistically controlled, the chance of delivering an LBW infant was more than twice as great for the women receiving Medicaid-financed care in private offices. The researchers attribute success of the health department's program to its greater emphasis on the use of ancillary services (e.g., home visiting and WIC) to supplement basic obstetric medical care.[5]

• In Washington State, increases in low birth weight among the poor have been linked to the economic recession of 1982 and concomitant restrictions on Medicaid eligibility.[9]

• Research among an indigent population in Texas shows that LBW infants whose mothers received comprehensive prenatal care had significantly lower perinatal morbidity and mortality than infants whose mothers received no prenatal care. Thus, prenatal care appears to affect both the incidence and the outcome of low weight births.[24]

Risk Factors

Key factors clearly associated with increased risk of LBW are race, age of mother (less than 18 or greater than 35), educational attainment of mother (risk decreases as educational status increases), low socioeconomic status, inadequate prenatal care, maternal smoking, maternal consumption of alcohol, birth order (risk increases for first births and for fourth or higher birth order), and marital status of mother (risk increases for out-of-wedlock births). In addition, recent evidence suggests that the risk of bearing an LBW infant is increased for women who continue stressful or strenuous employment outside the home in late pregnancy.[6, 13, 21, 26, 31, 42, 44, 46]

U.S. Objectives for Reducing the LBW Rate

In 1980, the U.S. Department of Health and Human Services set the following objectives for reducing the proportion of LBW babies born in the United States:

• By 1990, low birth weight babies should constitute no more than 5% of all live births.
• By 1990, no county and no racial or ethnic group of the population should have a rate of low birth weight infants that exceeds 9% of all live births.[37]

In a 1985 report to Congress, the Department of Health and Human Services projected that the United States will not meet the goal for the nation as a whole, nor will the goal for racial groups be reached for black infants. State-by-state analyses indicated that by 1990—

• 38 states will have LBW rates above 5% and
• of the 28 states that had more than 2,500 black births in 1978, only Kentucky will have a LBW rate that does not exceed 9%.[27]

Data Sources

State and Local

The most timely state and local data are available from each state's bureau of vital statistics (usually within the state's health department), which is responsible for collecting birth certificate data that will eventually be sent to the National Center for Health Statistics (NCHS). Most states publish birth data annually, including information on LBW infants. All states now link birth and death certificates, either by computer or manually. Some use the linked birth-death records to tabulate birth-weight specific infant mortality. Some states provide birth statistics by census tract. These data can be related to data on socioeconomic status, also available by census tract.

In large cities, the city or county health department (vital statistics registrar) may publish data on low birth weight. Smaller cities tend to rely on state publication of data.

Another source of state data on LBW is the NCHS publication *Advance Report of Final Natality Statistics,* part of the Monthly Vital Statistics Report series. The *Advance Report* provides the most recent LBW rates for each state by race.

The Children's Defense Fund is another source of state and local data on low birth weight. Its annual publication *The Health of America's Children: Maternal and Child Health Data Book* provides a wealth of information, including a ranking of states by their LBW rates (total, white, black, and nonwhite); a similar ranking of cities with populations greater than 500,000; and a year-by-year listing of states' LBW rates (by race) starting in 1978, with analysis of each state's progress toward meeting the Surgeon General's 1990 Objectives for the Nation.

National

National data on LBW are available from the NCHS Vital Statistics Registration System (VSRS), which continuously collects and compiles data from birth certificates. The VSRS provides data on LBW infants tabulated by race and sex of infant, and by mother's age, educational attainment, marital status, receipt of prenatal care, and interval since last birth. Data from the VSRS are published annually in an abbreviated form in the *Advance Report of Final Natality Statistics.* There is a one- to two-year lag between the end of a calendar year and publication of *Advance Report* data for that year. More complete but less timely data (three- to four-year lag) are available in another annual NCHS publication, *Vital Statistics of the United States, Vol. 1, Natality.*

The Children's Defense Fund publication *The Health of America's Children: Maternal and Child Health Data Book* is another source of annual data on LBW. This publication includes discussion of national progress in meeting the Surgeon General's 1990 Objectives for LBW; trend data on the U.S. LBW rate by race; and an international ranking of LBW rates.

The National Natality Surveys (NNS), conducted by NCHS in 1963–69, 1972, and 1980, provide periodic data on low birth weight by characteristics beyond those covered on birth certificates, such as mother's occupation and work history during pregnancy, father's occupation, source of medical care for mother and infant, family income, and mother's smoking and drinking habits. Data from the NNS are periodically available in a variety of publications, including reports in the Vital and Health Statistics series and supplements to the Monthly Vital Statistics Report series. Data from the 1980 NNS have been analyzed in a broad range of papers and publications, most of which are available from the Natality Branch of NCHS.[36] Public-use data tapes of the follow-back surveys are available from the National Technical Information Service (NTIS). Data collection for the next NNS, the National Maternal and Infant Health Survey, began in the fall of 1988 and will continue through 1990. It includes data on causes of LBW, the effects of maternal smoking and drug and alcohol use on pregnancy outcome, and methods used to prevent prematurity, as well as an evaluation of WIC, Medicaid, and other public programs serving pregnant women and infants.

Both the CDC and NCHS have recently initiated projects that evaluate linked birth-death certificate data. The CDC's National Infant Mortality Surveillance Project (NIMS) compiled the states' linked birth-death records to analyze data for the 1980 birth cohort. Findings have been reported in a special section of *Public Health Reports*.[38] Additional state-specific data from NIMS will be published and will be available on public-use data tapes in the future. The Linked Birth and Infant Death Record Project of NCHS is currently funded to link and analyze birth-death certificate data for the 1983–86 birth cohorts. It is anticipated that, starting with the 1987 birth cohort, this much-needed national data base will become part of routine data collection and reporting by NCHS. Public-use data tapes for the 1983 birth cohort should be available by March 1989. Tapes and publications for subsequent birth cohorts will be available in the future.

Data Needs

National

Perhaps the greatest problem with our national LBW data system has been the absence of ongoing national data on outcomes for LBW infants. To date, no national data system has regularly assessed the relationship between birth weight and subsequent morbidity, but the Linked Birth and Infant Death Record Project of NCHS is likely to fill this gap.

A second shortcoming of the current national data system is the considerable time lag between the end of a calendar year and publication of final national data for that year. There is a lag of approximately one to four years before publication of final VSRS data on LBW. In addition, it is projected that national linked birth-death certificate data for any given birth cohort may not be available until approximately four years after the year of birth. This relatively long lag makes it difficult to use timely national LBW data in evaluating, planning, and implementing public policies.

National LBW data by income (or class, as the British use) are very limited. Although the NNS does provide periodic data by income, the VSRS does not collect information by income or clear class ranking. As a result, surrogate measures such as race or mother's education are often used, making it more difficult to distinguish to what extent LBW is associated with poverty as distinct from other factors.

Although the NNS collects information from married mothers on sources of family income, including participation in public programs, there is no national data base that systematically and continuously links LBW data (incidence and outcome) to participation in public programs such as WIC, Medicaid, food stamps, and AFDC. This information, if linked with data on income or class, would be particularly useful in evaluating the impact of public policies and programs.

Finally, national data by ethnicity are less complete than they might be. The NNS does collect detailed ethnicity data, which are available on public-use data tapes; however, the NNS is conducted relatively infrequently. Although the VSRS currently collects data by ethnicity, reporting by states is uneven. National data on births of Hispanic parentage were first available for the 1978 cohort, based on reporting from 17 states. The 1985 data on Hispanics are based on reporting from 23 states and the District of Columbia.[49] Low birth weight data on births of Asian parentage (Chinese, Filipino, Japanese, Hawaiian, and other) were first published by NCHS in 1984.[45]

References

1. Baldwin W. Half empty, half full: what we know about low birth weight among blacks. JAMA 1986;255(3 Jan):86–8.

2. Behrman R. Premature births among black women. N Engl J Med 1987;317(17 Sep):763–5.

3. Binsacca D, Ellis J, Martin D, Pettitti D. Factors associated with low birthweight in an inner-city population: the role of financial problems. Am J Public Health 1987;77(Apr):505–6.

4. Brown S. Can low birth weight be prevented? Fam Plann Perspect 1985;17(May–Jun):112–8.

5. Buescher P, Smith C, Holliday J, Levine R. Source of prenatal care and infant birth weight: the case of a North Carolina county. Am J Obstet Gynecol 1987;156(Jan):204–10.

6. Council on Scientific Affairs. Effects of pregnancy on work performance. JAMA 1984; 251(20 Apr):1995–7.

7. David R. Did low birthweight among US blacks really increase? Am J Public Health 1986;76(Apr):380–3.

8. Endozien J, Switzer B, Bryan R. Medical evaluation of the Special Supplemental Food Program for Women, Infants and Children. Am J Clin Nutr 1979;32(Mar):677–92.

9. Fisher E, LoGerfo J, Daling J. Prenatal care and pregnancy outcomes during the recession: the Washington State experience. Am J Public Health 1985;75(Aug):866–9.

10. Hackman E, Emanuel I, van Belle G, Daling J. Maternal birth weight and subsequent pregnancy outcome. JAMA 1983;250(21 Oct):2016–9.

11. Hardy J, Drage J, Jackson E. The first year of life. Report from the Collaborative Perinatal Project of the National Institute of Neurological and Communicative Disorders and Stroke. Baltimore, MD: Johns Hopkins University Press, 1979.

12. Heckler M. Report of the Secretary's Task Force on Black and Minority Health. Vol 1, Executive summary. Washington, DC: U.S. Department of Health and Human Services, 1985.

13. Hemminki E, Starfield B. Prevention of low birth weight and pre-term birth. Milbank Mem Fund Q 1978;56(3):339–61.

14. Hughes D, Johnson K, Rosenbaum S, Butler E, Simons J. The health of America's children: maternal and child health data book. Washington, DC: Children's Defense Fund, 1988.

15. Hughes D, Johnson K, Rosenbaum S, Simons J, Butler E. The health of America's children: maternal and child health data book. Washington, DC: Children's Defense Fund, 1987.

16. Hunter R, Kilstrom N, Kraybill E, Loda F. Antecedents of child abuse and neglect in premature infants: a prospective study in a newborn intensive care unit. Pediatrics 1978;61(4):629–35.

17. Institute of Medicine. Preventing low birthweight. Washington, DC: National Academy Press, 1985.

18. Klein M, Stern L. Low birth weight and the battered child syndrome. Am J Dis Child 1971;122(Jul):15–8.

19. Kleinman J. The recent decline in infant mortality. In: Health—United States, 1980. DHHS Pub. No. (PHS)81–1232. Washington, DC: National Center for Health Statistics, 1980: 29–33.

20. Kleinman J. Trends and variations in birth weight. In: Health—United States, 1981. DHHS Pub. No. (PHS)82–1232. Washington, DC: National Center for Health Statistics, 1981: 7–13.

21. Kleinman J, Kessel S. Racial differences in low birth weight: trends and risk factors. N Engl J Med 1987;317(Sep):749–53.

22. Kleinman J, Madans J. The effects of maternal smoking, physical stature, and educational attainment on the incidence of low birth weight. Am J Epidemiol 1985;121(6):843–55.

23. Kotelchuck M, et al. WIC participation and pregnancy outcomes: Massachusetts Statewide Evaluation Study. Am J Public Health 1984;74(10):1145–9.

24. Leveno K, Cunningham G, Roark M, Nelson S, Williams M. Prenatal care and the low birth weight infant. Obstet Gynecol 1985;66(Nov):599–605.

25. Lieberman E, Ryan K, Monson R, Schoenbaum S. Risk factors accounting for racial differences in the rate of premature birth. N Engl J Med 1987;317(Sep):743–8.

26. Mamelle N, Laumon B, Lazar P. Prematurity and occupational activity during pregnancy. Am J Epidemiol 1984;119(3):309–22.

27. Mason J. Report to the Subcommittee on Oversight and Investigation of the Committee on Energy and Commerce, U.S. House of Representatives, 3 Apr. Washington, DC: Department of Health and Human Services, 1985.

28. McCormick M. The contribution of low birth weight to infant mortality and childhood morbidity. N Engl J Med 1985;312(10 Jan):82–90.

29. Miller J. Sickle cell trait in pregnancy. S Med J 1983;76(8):962–3.

30. Naeye R. Causes of the excessive rates of perinatal mortality and prematurity in pregnancies complicated by maternal urinary tract infections. N Engl J Med 1979;300:(15)819–23.

31. Naeye R, Peters E. Working during pregnancy: effects on the fetus. Pediatrics 1982;69(Jun):724–7.

32. National Center for Health Statistics. Vital statistics of the United States, 1975. Vol 1, Natality. DHHS Pub. No. (PHS)78–1113. Washington, DC: NCHS, 1978.

33. National Center for Health Statistics. Health—United States, 1983. DHHS Pub. No. (PHS)84–1232. Washington, DC: NCHS, 1983.

34. National Center for Health Statistics. Advance report of final natality statistics, 1985. Monthly Vital Statistics Report 36(4). Supplement. DHHS Pub. No. (PHS)87–1120. Washington, DC: NCHS, 1987.

35. National Center for Health Statistics. Vital statistics of the United States, 1985. Vol 1, Natality. DHHS Pub. No. (PHS)87–1113. Washington, DC: NCHS, 1987.

36. Placek P. One hundred and twenty-five (125) reports, papers, and publications using the 1980 Natality Survey and the 1980 National Fetal Mortality Survey. Washington, DC: National Center for Health Statistics, 1987.

37. Public Health Service. Promoting health/preventing disease: objectives for the nation. DHHS Pub. No. (OM)81–0007. Washington, DC: PHS, 1980.

38. Public Health Service. Special section—National surveillance of infant mortality. Public Health Reports 1987;102(Mar–Apr):126–216.

39. Richmond J, Filner B. Infant and child health: needs and strategies. In: Healthy people: the Surgeon General's report on health promotion and disease prevention. Background Papers. DHEW Pub. No. (PHS)79–55071A. Washington, DC: PHS, 1979.

40. Shiono P, Klebanoff M, Graubard B, Berendes H, Rhoads G. Birth weight among women of different ethnic groups. JAMA 1986;255(3 Jan):48–52.

41. Shotland J. Rising poverty, declining health: the nutritional status of the rural poor. Washington, DC: Public Voice for Food and Health Policy, 1986.

42. Showstack J, Budetti P, Minkler D. Factors associated with birthweight: an exploration of the roles of prenatal care and length of gestation. Am J Public Health 1984;74(Sep):1003–8.

43. Stockbauer J. WIC prenatal participation and its relation to pregnancy outcomes in Missouri: a second look. Am J Public Health 1987;77(Jul):813–8.

44. Taffel S. Factors associated with low birth weight: United States, 1976. DHEW Pub. No. (PHS)80–1915. Washington, DC: National Center for Health Statistics, 1980.

45. Taffel S. Characteristics of Asian births: United States, 1980. Monthly Vital Statistics Report 32(10). Supplement. DHHS Pub. No. (PHS)84–1120. Washington, DC: National Center for Health Statistics, 1984.

46. Terris M. The epidemiology of prematurity: studies of specific etiologic factors. In: Chipman S, Lillienfeld A, Greenberg G, Donnelly J, eds. Research methodology and needs in perinatal studies. Springfield, IL: Charles C Thomas, 1966.

47. U.S. Department of Agriculture. Estimation of eligibility for the WIC program: report of the WIC Eligibility Study. Summary of Data, Method and Findings. USDA Contract No. 53-3198-3-138. Washington, DC: USDA, 1987.

48. Ventura S. Births of Hispanic parentage, 1983 and 1984. Monthly Vital Statistics Report 36(4). Supplement (2). DHHS Pub. No. (PHS)87-1120. Washington, DC: PHS, 1987.

49. Ventura S. Births of Hispanic heritage, 1988. Monthly Vital Statistics Report 36(11). Supplement. DHHS Pub. No. (PHS)88-1120. Washington, DC: PHS, 1988.

50. Ventura S, Taffel S. Childbearing characteristics of U.S.- and foreign-born Hispanic mothers. Public Health Reports 1985;100(Nov–Dec):647-52.

Infant Mortality Rate

Indicators

- The number of deaths to infants under one year of age per 1,000 live births (infant mortality rate).
- The number of deaths to infants under 28 days per 1,000 live births (neonatal mortality rate).
- The number of deaths to infants aged 28 days to one year per 1,000 live births (postneonatal mortality rate).

Significance

Policy and Program Implications

The infant mortality rate (IMR) is generally regarded as a quality of life indicator of both the health and welfare of a population. Disparities among population groups reflect differences in access to adequate food, shelter, education, sanitation, and health care.

Neonatal mortality tends to be closely associated with low birth weight and with influences occurring prenatally, during birth, and in the newborn period—such as poor maternal nutrition and health habits, lack of high-quality obstetric and neonatal health services, and congenital defects not compatible with life. Postneonatal mortality generally tends to be associated with environmental circumstances for the infant, particularly those linked to poverty—such as inadequate food or sanitation, unsafe housing, lack of health services, and inadequate supervision.

Status and Trends

National

In 1985, a total of 40,030 infants in the U.S. died before reaching their first birthdays. With an IMR of 10.6 deaths per 1,000 live births, American infants fared worse than those in 17 other nations.[31, 45]

- A review of maternal and infant health in western Europe found that countries with fewer resources than the United States are doing a better job of preventing infant mortality. Key elements in the European approach to infant mortality are readily available provider systems, removal of economic and other barriers to the use of these systems, and linkage of prenatal care to comprehensive social and financial benefits.[28]

• Although the U.S. infant mortality rate for 1985 was lower than the rate for the 1984, the change was not statistically significant.[31]

• In the 1980s, the United States has experienced a slowing in the decline of the IMR, a reversal of the trend for the previous decade. During the 1970s, the IMR declined an average of 4.6% annually. In contrast, from 1981 to 1985, the average annual decline has been only 2.9%. The United States has not experienced this kind of plateauing of the IMR since the decade from 1955 to 1965.[7, 31] Analysts sometimes argue that a favorable trend slows as it approaches optimum levels, but this has not been the case with infant mortality in the United States. Slowing has been most pronounced among populations with the highest rates.

• Economic downswings, increasing poverty rates among women and children, reductions in and reorganization of publicly funded health care services, and the absence of health insurance of any kind for many of the working poor have all been linked to the recent plateau in infant mortality in the United States.[2, 8, 27, 38]

• Black infants born in this country die at amost twice the rate of white infants. In 1985, the IMR for blacks was 18.2 per 1,000 live births, compared with a rate of 9.3 for whites. The United States has experienced no significant improvement in this racial disparity over the past 25 years. In fact, in 1985, the ratio of black to white infant deaths was slightly higher than it was in 1960—1.95 versus 1.93.[17, 31]

• Neonatal deaths account for two-thirds of all infant deaths, with the majority of neonatal deaths occurring in the first week of life. As with infant mortality as a whole, the decline in the neonatal mortality rate has begun to slow in recent years.[13, 15, 23, 31]

• In 1985, for the first time in more than 25 years, the neonatal mortality rate in the United States failed to decline at all, remaining constant at 7.0 deaths per 1,000 live births. For blacks, the neonatal mortality rate increased between 1984 and 1985 from 11.8 to 12.1 deaths per 1,000 live births. This was the first increase in black neonatal mortality since 1964. White neonatal mortality declined slightly between 1984 and 1985 from 6.2 to 6.1 deaths per 1,000 live births. (For both blacks and whites, the changes between 1984 and 1985 were not statistically significant.)[17, 31]

• Although neonatal mortality has declined for both blacks and whites over the past 25 years, it has declined more rapidly for whites. As a result, the ratio of black to white neonatal mortality rates has increased from 1.62 in 1960 to 1.98 in 1985.[17, 31]

- The racial gap in neonatal mortality reflects both a higher incidence of low birth weight among blacks and a poorer survival rate for black infants weighing 3,000 g or more.[3, 15, 36]

- Reductions in the neonatal mortality rate since the mid-1960s have been closely linked to the improved survival of low birth weight babies, generally attributed to better obstetric and pediatric management during labor, delivery, and the neonatal period.[10, 11, 19] However, at least part of the decline in neonatal mortality can be attributed to the fact that fewer high-risk infants are born, because of better access to prenatal care, as well as to family planning and abortion services.[6, 12, 19, 23, 44] Recent research identifies abortion, improved schooling for women, WIC, and Medicaid as program determinants that may have had at least as great an impact in reducing neonatal mortality as neonatal intensive care.[5]

- Postneonatal mortality has declined substantially since the 1960s. However, progress has not been steady, and the rate of decline has slowed in recent years. Since 1970, the postneonatal mortality rate has seen year-to-year increases in 1975, 1978, and 1983. The 1985 rate was 3.7 deaths per 1,000 live births, compared with a rate of 3.8 in 1984.[17, 20, 31]

- The racial gap in postneonatal mortality has narrowed over the past 25 years; however, substantial disparities remain. In 1960, black infants were nearly three times as likely as white infants to die during the postneonatal period. In 1985, the ratio of black to white postneonatal deaths was 2 to 1.[17, 31]

- Between 1970 and 1985, the relative contribution of postneonatal deaths to total infant mortality rose from 25% to 35%. This increase should prompt a closer look at policies and programs associated with reductions in postneonatal mortality. Recent research links increases in the availability of federally funded community health centers with decreases in postneonatal mortality rates and with a lessening of racial disparities in these rates. Additionally, higher federal expenditures for health care services and higher pediatrician-to-infant ratios have been linked to reductions in postneonatal deaths.[31, 43]

- An evaluation of the WIC program (Special Supplemental Food Program for Women, Infants, and Children) indicates that it contributed significantly to the reduction of infant mortality.[22]

- Programs such as Maternal and Infant Care and community health centers might have had a more impressive national impact on infant mortality if a higher proportion of eligible women had been reached by these programs. Evidence is strong that among local populations who in fact were reached, the outcomes improved greatly.[41]

• Efforts that significantly reduce the occurrence of low birth weight are likely to have a greater impact on the overall infant mortality rate than are additional investments in medical care designed to save babies who are born too soon or too small.[4, 14, 25, 26, 37] Additionally, disparities in the IMR suggest the need for tailoring preventive services to meet the varied and special needs of high-risk populations.[46]

State and Local

• The risk of infant mortality varies considerably by state and region. Using a four-region division of the states, the Centers for Disease Control (CDC) analyzed infant mortality data for the 1980 birth cohort. The region with the highest infant mortality risk (number of infant deaths per 1,000 live births in the birth cohort) was the South (12.1), followed by the North Central Region (10.8), the Northeast (10.4), and the West (9.9). Although a significant portion (72%) of the excess mortality in the South can be attributed to a higher proportion of black births, black infants actually fared better in the South (infant mortality risk of 18.6) than they did in either the North Central Region (20.7) or the Northeast (19.0). In contrast, white infants fared significantly worse in the South than in the rest of the nation. This higher infant mortality risk for Southern whites contributed 28% of excess infant deaths in the region.[1]

• In 1985, 7 of the 10 states with the highest IMRs for all races combined were Southern; however, only 3 of the 10 states with the highest black IMRs were located in the South.[16]

• CDC analysts report that black infants fare significantly better in the West than in the remainder of the country. If black infants throughout the country experienced the same infant mortality risk as those in the West, black infant mortality risk in the United States would decrease by 13%. The lower black infant mortality risk in the West can be attributed to both a smaller proportion of LBW infants and a lower birth weight–specific mortality, both of which can be affected by quality and availability of medical care. These findings suggest that improvement in the survival of black infants is attainable and point to the need for policies and programs that improve prenatal, perinatal, and infant care among this high-risk population.[1]

• In 1985, the District of Columbia had a higher IMR than any state (20.8), followed by Delaware (14.8) and South Carolina (14.2). Rhode

Island had the lowest IMR (8.2), followed by Vermont, Nevada, and North Dakota (all at 8.5).[16]

• Between 1984 and 1985, 17 states experienced increases in their total IMRs; 18 experienced increases for whites and 17 saw increases for nonwhites. Of the 32 states with large enough black populations to provide reliable data, 12 experienced an increase in the black IMR. States with particularly large increases between 1984 and 1985 are: Delaware (37% increase for all infants, 38% for whites, and 33% for blacks), Massachusetts (46% increase for blacks), and Oklahoma (25% increase for blacks).[16]

• The National Center for Health Statistics (NCHS) reports that from 1981 through 1983, eight states and the District of Columbia had IMRs more than 5% above the national average. These states were Florida, Illinois, Indiana, Kentucky, Michigan, Oklahoma, Pennsylvania, and South Carolina.[21]

• In Kentucky, poor infants are more than twice as likely as nonpoor infants to die during the postneonatal period. Based on infant deaths from 1982 to 1983, researchers calculate that approximately half of 201 postneonatal deaths among poor infants were "preventable"—that is, they would not have occurred if the babies had not been born into poverty. The researchers call for efforts to reduce the number of families living in poverty and for a governmental commitment to assure access to health services throughout the postneonatal period.[42]

• In 1983, the infant mortality rate for rural low-income counties was 46.4% higher than for the rest of the nation. This gap increased by 32% between 1981 and 1983.[40]

• In 1985, among U.S. cities with populations greater than 500,000, the District of Columbia had the highest IMR for all races combined (20.8). For whites, New York City had the highest IMR (13.8), and for blacks, Boston's IMR was highest (25.3).[16]

• Between 1968 and 1981, the District of Columbia experienced essentially no change in its IMR for nonwhites. Among cities with populations over 500,000, the District has the third highest IMR for blacks and the seventh highest for nonwhites.[16, 21]

• In Los Angeles between 1984 and 1985, the county IMR rose from 9.8 to 10.4 deaths per 1,000 live births—the first increase in over a decade. County health officials link this rise to the county's inability to provide enough prenatal services to keep pace with a rapid increase in births.[32]

- In 1986, Chicago's IMR was 16.5 deaths per 1,000 live births, significantly higher than the rate for the state as a whole (11.6). The IMR in Chicago appears to have plateaued, showing virtually no change for three years in a row. The record for postneonatal mortality is worse, remaining virtually constant for five years in a row. Black infants in Chicago die at almost twice the rate of white infants, and in the postneonatal period the black-to-white mortality ratio is nearly 3 to 1. Chicago's Commissioner of Public Health cites several factors contributing to the city's high infant death rate, including long-term limitations in Medicaid coverage in the state, lack of any medical coverage for many of the city's working poor, inadequate funding for public sector health care providers, maldistribution of health care resources within the city, limitations of recent state efforts to reimburse perinatal centers for care of public aid recipients, and the unrelenting stresses of poverty affecting a high proportion of Chicago's pregnant women and infants.[8]

- A Harvard University study of infant deaths in five Boston neighborhoods found that the IMR rose 46% between 1981 and 1982. Neonatal mortality increased 58% in the same year. The study relates the dramatic increase in deaths to a drop in essential health care services formerly funded by the federal government—specifically, cuts in funding for the Maternal and Child Health Program and reduced eligibility for Medicaid.[9]

Risk Factors

The following are risk factors most commonly measured and found to be associated with infant mortality in the United States today:
- for the infant—low birth weight, congenital defects, inadequate intrapartum and neonatal care, high birth order, and race (increased for black infants).
- for the mother—under age 18 or over age 35, previous fetal or infant loss, poor health prior to or during the pregnancy, inadequate prenatal nutrition, low socioeconomic status, low educational attainment, smoking, and substance abuse.[11, 18, 19, 23, 39, 46]

U.S. Objectives for Reducing Infant Mortality

In 1980, the U.S. Department of Health and Human Services set the following objectives for reducing the IMR in the United States:
- By 1990, the national IMR should be reduced to no more than 9 deaths per 1,000 live births.
- By 1990, no county and no racial or ethnic group of the population should have an IMR in excess of 12 deaths per 1,000 live births.

- By 1990, the neonatal death rate should be reduced to no more than 6.5 deaths per 1,000 live births.[34]

In a 1985 report to Congress, the Department of Health and Human Services projected that the United States will meet the overall goal of no more than 9 infant deaths per 1,000 live births. However, the nation will not meet the goal of 12 deaths per 1,000 live births for blacks. Further projections by the department indicate that in 1990—

- 12 states will have IMRs above 9 and
- of the 28 states that had more than 2,500 black births in 1978, 21 will have IMRs above 12.[24]

Data Sources

State and Local

The most timely state and local data on infant mortality are available from each state's registrar of vital statistics (usually in the state's department of health). Most states publish mortality data annually. All states now link birth and death certificates, either by computer or manually. Some use the linked birth-death records to tabulate infant deaths by factors such as receipt of prenatal care; birth weight; and mother's age, educational status, and occupation. Some states can provide infant mortality data by census tract. These data can be related to data on socioeconomic status, also available by census tract.

In large cities, the city or county health department may publish data on infant deaths. Smaller cities tend to rely on state publication of data.

Another source of data for states and localities is the NCHS report *Vital Statistics of the United States, Vol. II, Mortality*. It annually reports the total number of infant deaths for states, metropolitan areas (SMSAs), counties, and selected cities with populations over 10,000. The state data are tabulated by race and cause of death. Data for localities are tabulated by cause of death only. NCHS also publishes a much shorter but more timely publication, *Advance Report of Final Mortality Statistics*, which includes a listing of infant and neonatal deaths and death rates by state.

The Children's Defense Fund, a private nonprofit organization based in Washington, DC, annually publishes *The Health of America's Children: Maternal and Child Health Data Book*. This publication provides a wealth of information, including a ranking of states by their infant, neonatal, and postneonatal mortality rates (total, white, black, and nonwhite); a similar ranking of cities with populations greater than 500,000; and a year-by-year listing of states' infant, neonatal, and postneonatal mortality rates (by race) over an eight-year period, with analysis of each state's progress toward meeting the Surgeon General's 1990 Objectives for the Nation.

National

National data on the incidence of infant mortality (including neonatal and postneonatal deaths) are available from the NCHS Vital Statistics Registration System (VSRS), which continuously collects and compiles data from death certificates. The VSRS provides data on the incidence of infant mortality tabulated by cause of death (including the 10 leading causes of infant death), age, sex, race, and national origin of the infant. Data from the VSRS are published annually in an abbreviated form in the *Advance Report of Final Mortality Statistics,* part of the NCHS Monthly Vital Statistics Report series. There is about a two-year lag between the end of a calendar year and publication of *Advance Report* data for that year. More complete, but less timely data (about a three-year lag) are available in another annual NCHS publication, *Vital Statistics of the United States, Vol. II, Mortality.*

Another annual source of national data is the Children's Defense Fund publication *The Health of America's Children: Maternal and Child Health Data Book,* which includes information on national progress in meeting the Surgeon General's 1990 Objectives for infant, neonatal, and postneonatal mortality (by race); international rankings of national IMRs; and a year-by-year listing by race of the national IMR (from 1940) and neonatal and postneonatal mortality rates (from 1950).

Periodic data on infant mortality are available from a series of special studies conducted by NCHS: the National Linked Birth-Infant Death Records Study of Infant Mortality,[30] the National Infant Mortality Follow-Back Survey,[29] and the National Natality Survey/National Death Index Match.[33] These studies report on infant deaths tabulated by characteristics such as mother's age, educational status, and employment; receipt of prenatal care; household composition; income; father's occupation; health insurance; and hospitalization of the infant who died.

Both the CDC and NCHS have undertaken projects that evaluate linked birth-death certificate data. The CDC's National Infant Mortality Surveillance Project (NIMS) compiled the states' linked birth-death records to analyze data for the 1980 birth cohort. Findings have been reported in a special section of *Public Health Reports.*[35] Additional state-specific data from NIMS will be published and will be available on public-use data tapes in the future. The Linked Birth and Infant Death Record Project of NCHS is currently funded to link and analyze birth-death certificate data for the 1983–86 birth cohorts. Public-use data tapes for the 1983 birth cohort should be available in spring 1989. Tapes and publications for subsequent birth cohorts will be available in the future. It is anticipated that, starting with the 1987 birth cohort, this much-needed national data base will become part of routine data collection and reporting by NCHS.

Data Needs

State and Local

In response to the general slowing of the decline in the IMR, the Public Health Service has assembled a cadre of health professionals to provide expert assistance to states to conduct infant mortality reviews and investigations of conditions associated with high or changing infant mortality. The approach is designed to assist state health departments in gaining a better understanding of the nature of local difficulties in reducing infant mortality. It is also aimed at gathering precise information concerning local maternal and infant health care systems and opportunities for improvement.

National

Perhaps the greatest gap in our national data base has been the absence of an ongoing system linking infant birth-death certificate data. It has been necessary to rely on infrequent special studies to evaluate the relationship between infant mortality and specific maternal and infant characteristics such as low birth weight or mother's receipt of prenatal care. At long last, it appears that linked birth-death records are soon to become part of the national data system: The Linked Birth and Infant Death Record Project of NCHS is currently funded to cover four birth cohorts, and it is anticipated that ongoing funding will be obtained so that the project can become a part of routine data collection and reporting by the VSRS.

A second shortcoming of the current national data system is the time lag between the end of a calendar year and publication of final national data. NCHS has been successful in shortening the lag in recent years and continues to make this a priority; however, it still takes approximately two to three years before publication of final VSRS data on infant mortality. In addition, it is projected that national linked birth-death certificate data for any given birth cohort would not be available until approximately four years after the year of birth. For purposes of evaluating, planning, and implementing public policies, the longer the lag, the more difficult it is to use national infant mortality data in a timely manner.

National infant mortality data by income (or class, as the British use) are very limited. Although the National Infant Mortality Follow-Back Surveys do provide periodic data by income, the VSRS does not collect information by income or clear class ranking. As a result, surrogate measures such as race or mother's education are often used, making it more difficult to distinguish to what extent infant mortality is associated with poverty as distinct from other factors.

There is no ongoing national data base that systematically links infant mortality data with participation in public programs such as WIC, Medicaid, food stamps, and AFDC. This information, if linked with data on income or class, would be particularly useful in evaluating the impact of public policies and programs.

Finally, national data by ethnicity and racial group other than white and black are less complete than they might be. Although NCHS does currently collect data by ethnicity, reporting by states is quite uneven. NCHS does not currently publish data on infant mortality among Hispanics; however, Hispanic IMRs are available from the Mortality Branch. Infant mortality data for American Indian, Chinese, and Japanese populations are published annually in a single table in *Vital Statistics of the United States, Vol. II, Mortality.*

References

1. Allen D, Buehler J, Hogue C, Strauss L, Smith J. Regional differences in birth weight-specific infant mortality, United States, 1980. Public Health Reports 1987;102(Mar–Apr): 138–45.

2. American Academy of Pediatrics. Task Force on Infant Mortality: statement on infant mortality. Pediatrics 1986;78(Dec):1155–60.

3. Binkin N, Williams R, Hogue C, Chen P. Reducing black neonatal mortality: will improvement in birth weight be enough? JAMA 1985;253(18 Jan):372–5.

4. Buehler J, Kleinman J, Hogue C, Strauss L, Smith J. Birth weight–specific infant mortality, United States, 1960 and 1980. Public Health Reports 1987;102(Mar–Apr):151–61.

5. Corman H, Grossman M. Determinants of neonatal mortality rates in the United States: a reduced form model. Working Paper No. 1387. Cambridge, MA: National Bureau of Economic Research, 1984.

6. David R, Siegel E. Decline in neonatal mortality, 1968–1977: better babies or better care? Report from a Northwestern U./U. of North Carolina joint project. Chicago: Children's Memorial Hospital, 1983.

7. Division of Maternal and Child Health. Effective pregnancy and infant care—an initiative to reduce infant mortality in the United States. Washington, DC: U.S. Public Health Service, Department of Health and Human Services, 1984.

8. Edwards L. Testimony before the Select Committee on Children, Youth, and Families, U.S. House of Representatives, 5 Oct 1987. Chicago.

9. Feldman P. Preserving essential services: effects of the Maternal and Child Health Block Grants on local funding. Executive Summary. Boston: Harvard University, 1984.

10. Goldenberg R, Humphrey J, Hale C, Boyd B, Wayne J. Neonatal deaths in Alabama, 1979–1980: an analysis of birth weight- and race-specific neonatal mortality rates. Am J Obstet Gynecol 1983;145(1 Mar):545–52.

11. Goldenberg R, Humphrey J, Hale C, Wayne J, Boyd B. Neonatal mortality in Alabama 1970–1980. J Med Assoc State Ala 1982;(Aug):6–8,13

12. Grossman M, Jacobowitz S. Variations in infant mortality rates among counties of the United States: the roles of public policies and programs. In: van der Gaag J, Neenan W, Tsukahara T, Jr, eds. Economics of health care. New York: Praeger, 1982: 272–301.

13. Heckler M. Report of the Secretary's Task Force on Black and Minority Health. Vol 1, Executive summary. Washington, DC: U.S. Department of Health and Human Services, 1985.

14. Hemminki E, Starfield B. Prevention of low birth weight and pre-term birth. Milbank Mem Fund Q 1978;56(3):339–61.

15. Hogue C, Buehler J. Strauss L, Smith J. Overview of the National Infant Mortality Surveillance Project. Public Health Reports 1987;102(Mar–Apr):126–37.

16. Hughes D, Johnson K, Rosenbaum S, Butler E, Simons J. The health of America's children: maternal and child health data book. Washington, DC: Children's Defense Fund, 1988.

17. Hughes D, Johnson K, Rosenbaum S, Simons J, Butler E. The health of America's children: maternal and child health data book. Washington, DC: Children's Defense Fund, 1987.

18. Kessner D. Contrasts in health status. Vol 1, Infant death: an analysis by maternal risk and health care. Washington, DC: National Academy of Sciences, 1973.

19. Kleinman J. The recent decline in infant mortality. In: Health—United States, 1980. DHHS Pub. No. (PHS)81–1232. Washington, DC: National Center for Health Statistics, 1980:29–33.

20. Kleinman J. Tables on infant, neonatal and postneonatal mortality data. Washington, DC: Office of Statistical Resources, Mortality Branch, National Center for Health Statistics, 1985.

21. Kleinman J. State trends in infant mortality, 1968–1983. Am J Public Health 1986;76(Jun):681–8.

22. Kotelchuck M, et al. WIC participation and pregnancy outcomes: Massachusetts WIC Evaluation.. Am J. Public Health 1984;74(10):1086–92.

23. Kovar M. Pregnancy and childbirth. In: Better health for our children: a national strategy; vol. 3, Report of the Select Panel for the Promotion of Child Health. DHHS Pub. No. (PHS)79–55071. Washington, DC: PHS, 1981.

24. Mason J. Report to the Subcommittee on Oversight and Investigation, Committee on Energy and Commerce, U.S. House of Representatives, 3 Apr. Washington, DC: Department of Health and Human Services, 1985.

25. McCormick M. The contribution of low birth weight to infant mortality and childhood morbidity. N Engl J Med 1985;312(10 Jan):82–90.

26. McCormick M, Shapiro S, Starfield B. The regionalization of perinatal services; summary of the evaluation of a national demonstration program. JAMA 1985;253(8 Feb):799–804.

27. Miller C. Infant mortality in the U.S. Sci Am 1985;253(1):31–7.

28. Miller C. Maternal and infant survival. Washington, DC: National Center for Clinical Infant Programs, 1987.

29. National Center for Health Statistics. Infant mortality rate: socioeconomic factors, United States. Vital and Health Statistics, Series 22, No. 14. DHEW Pub. No. (HSM)72–1045. Washington, DC: NCHS, 1972.

30. National Center for Health Statistics. A study of infant mortality from linked records, by birth weight, period of gestation, and other variables, United States. Vital and Health Statistics, Series 20, No. 12. DHEW Pub. No. (HSM)72–1055. Washington, DC: NCHS, 1972.

31. National Center for Health Statistics. Advance report of final mortality statistics, 1985. Monthly Vital Statistics Report 36(28 Aug). Supplement. DHHS Pub. No. (PHS)87–1120. Washington, DC: NCHS, 1987.

32. Nelson H. L.A. County's infant death rate appears on the rise. Los Angeles Times, 29 July 1987.

33. Placek P. One hundred and twenty-five (125) reports, papers, and publications using the 1980 Natality Survey and the 1980 National Fetal Mortality Survey. Washington, DC: National Center for Health Statistics, 1987.

34. Public Health Service. Promoting health/preventing disease: objectives for the nation. DHHS Pub. No. (OM)81–0007. Washington, DC: PHS, 1980.

35. Public Health Service. Special section—National surveillance of infant mortality. Public Health Reports 1987;102(Mar–Apr):126–216.

36. Sappenfield W, Buehler J, Binkin N, Hogue C, Strauss L, Smith J. Differences in neonatal and postneonatal mortality by race, birth weight, and gestational age. Public Health Reports 1987;102(Mar–Apr):182–91.

37. Shapiro S. New reductions in infant mortality: the challenge of low birthweight. Am J Public Health 1981;71(4):365–6.

38. Shapiro S. Socio-demographic risk factors in infant mortality and low birthweight. Paper presented at Health Policy Forum, Harvard School of Public Health, Boston, 15 Oct 1984.

39. Shapiro S, McCormick M, Starfield B, Krischer J, Bross D. Relevance of correlates of infant death for significant morbidity at a year of age. Am J Obstet Gynecol 1980;136(3):363–73.

40. Shotland J. Rising poverty, declining health: the nutritional status of the rural poor. Washington, DC: Public Voice for Food and Health Policy, 1986.

41. Sokol R, Woolf R, Rosen M, Weingarden K. Risk, antepartum care, and outcome: impact of a maternity and infant care project. Obstet Gynecol 1980;56(2):150–6.

42. Spurlock C, Hinds M, Skaggs J, Hernandez C. Infant death rates among the poor and nonpoor in Kentucky, 1982 to 1983. Pediatrics 1987;80(Aug):262–9.

43. Starfield B. Postneonatal mortality. Annual Review of Public Health 1985;6:21–40.

44. Wallace H, Goldstein H, Ericson A. Comparison of infant mortality in the United States and Sweden. Clin Pediatr 1982;21(Mar):156–62.

45. Wegman M. Annual summary of vital statistics—1986. Pediatrics 1987;80(6):817–27.

46. Wise P, Kotelchuck M, Wilson M, Mills M. Racial and socioeconomic disparities in childhood mortality in Boston. N Engl J Med 1985;313(6):360–6.

CHAPTER 3

Indicators of Special Importance to Children

Inadequate Immunization Status

Definition

Immunization status is a measurable indicator of nonsusceptibility to specific infectious diseases. Immunity to disease is the ability of an individual to resist infection and may be conferred through artificial immunization or through previous natural infection.

Indicator

- In a defined population, the percentage of children who are not fully immunized against vaccine- or toxoid-preventable childhood diseases—diphtheria, tetanus, pertussis, measles, mumps, rubella, and polio. Being fully immunized means having met recommended schedules for active immunization.[2]

Significance

Immunization status is not a health outcome; however, it is closely and indisputably linked to rates of childhood diseases and is a good short-term predictor of long-term changes in disease incidence. Hence, immunization rates for a population are a valid surrogate measure of health outcomes or disease rates. Immunization rates for two-year-old children serve as a proxy measure for the proportion of young children receiving well-child health care. High immunization rates for school-aged children reflect compliance with state laws requiring evidence of immunization at the time of first enrollment in school.

Health Implications

Because the infectious agents of the vaccine- or toxoid-preventable childhood diseases have not yet been eradicated, any decline in immunization rates can be expected to increase the risk of new outbreaks of these diseases, with an increase in unnecessary disability and death as a result. A marked nationwide fall in immunization rates could lead to local or widespread epidemics similar to those occurring prior to the introduction of mass immunization efforts.

A question arises as to what levels of immunity must be maintained to prevent outbreaks or epidemics of vaccine- or toxoid-preventable childhood diseases. That is, what is the minimum level necessary to maintain "herd immunity"? There is no simple answer. First, even when the immunity level of the general population is high, it is possible for outbreaks to occur among circumscribed unimmunized subpopulations. Second, in some cases, levels previously thought to afford community protection have been challenged. For example, although 70% immunity has generally been thought to be high enough to protect against diphtheria outbreaks, new evidence suggests that higher immunity levels may be necessary to offer protection in densely populated communities and against especially virulent strains of bacteria.[20] For some diseases (e.g., rubella), immunity levels of 85% to 90% may not be high enough to halt spread of infection. For still other diseases (e.g., tetanus, which is not communicable in humans), there is no herd immunity (i.e., 100% immunization is necessary to assure individual protection).[17]

Policy and Program Implications

The immunization status of a population reflects the community's commitment to preventive public health efforts. A fall in immunization rates may reflect a change in policy or program priorities, or it may indicate a decreased capacity of public health agencies to meet stated objectives.

Attention has focused on adverse reactions to vaccines as a possible deterrent to routine immunization. Pertussis vaccine is especially troublesome because of its occasional toxicity and incomplete effectiveness. One careful analysis of benefits, risks, and costs estimated that without an immunization program there would be a 71-fold increase in cases of pertussis and an almost fourfold increase in deaths (from 2.0 to 7.6 per cohort of 1 million children).[16]

Cost-Effectiveness

Despite the rising costs of vaccines, immunization programs save dollars and prevent disease, disability, and death. For every dollar spent on the Childhood Immunization Program, the government saves roughly $10 in medical costs and lost productivity.[15]

The use of vaccines in developed countries is known to be cost-effective against measles, mumps, and rubella in high-risk groups.[21] In 1983, the combined measles-mumps-rubella vaccination program saved $14.40 for every dollar spent on immunization.[22] In the 25 years since the measles vaccine's licensure, the United States has saved $5.1 billion in direct and indirect costs.

An estimate of the average lifetime cost of each case of congenital rubella is $200,000.[3] For 1 million two-year-olds, rubella vaccination would save $9.8 million in net medical costs and an additional $7.4 million in productivity.[1]

Status and Trends

National

• The percentage of fully immunized children varies by age group. According to the U.S. Immunization Survey (USIS), the five- to six-year-old population has historically enjoyed the highest recorded immunization rates. However, in 1985, the best rates generally were among five- to nine-year olds; in this group, roughly 10% were inadequately immunized for measles and mumps, 12% were inadequately immunized for rubella and polio, and only 6% were not fully immunized for DTP (diphtheria, tetanus, and pertussis) (Figure 1).[4]

• Also in 1985, the lowest immunization rates were among children ages one to four. In fact, the percentage of preschoolers not fully immunized was disturbingly high, with more than one child in five inadequately immunized for measles, mumps, rubella, and polio. The proportion of children not fully immunized was 11 to 16 percentage points higher among nonwhites than whites (Figure 2).[4]

• Immunization levels in large urban areas remain below the levels in other areas. Among all one- to four-year-olds living in large cities, approximately one-fourth did not receive measles, mumps, or rubella vaccine in 1985. Among nonwhite one- to four-year-olds living in big cities, approximately one-third were not vaccinated for measles, mumps, or rubella. Evidence suggests that the high proportion of unimmunized children in large cities reflects poor access to basic health services and that disparities between white and nonwhite children are linked to economic status (Figure 3).[4, 13]

• Following the initiation of a federal childhood immunization drive, the number of measles cases decreased from 13,597 in 1979 to an all-time low of 1,497 in 1983. However, increases in reported cases occurred in both 1984 (2,587) and 1985 (2,822). Data for 1986 indicate an alarming 6,282 cases of measles, a 2.2-fold increase over 1985. Children younger than age five accounted for 39% of these cases, with 7 of 10 cases among children ages 16 months to four years being preventable.[5] Sixty percent of all reported cases in 1986 were attributable to inadequate immunization status (Table 1).[5, 8]

• In 1985, reported cases of mumps reached an all-time low of 2,982. However, after 15 years of continual decline, the number escalated to 7,790 cases in 1986; two-thirds of the reported cases were among children under

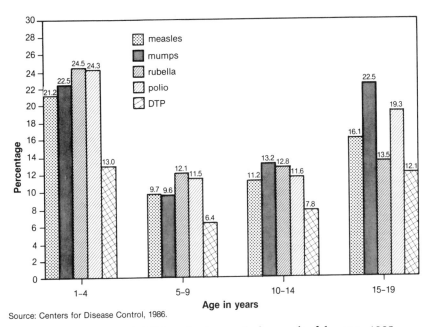

Source: Centers for Disease Control, 1986.

Figure 1. Percentage of children inadequately immunized by age, 1985.

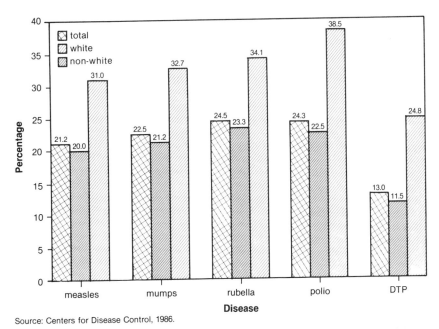

Source: Centers for Disease Control, 1986.

Figure 2. Percentage of one- to four-year-olds inadequately immunized by race, 1985.

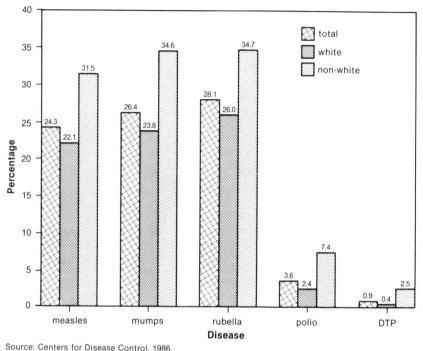

Source: Centers for Disease Control, 1986.

Figure 3. Percentage of one- to four-year-olds who received no vaccine in big cities by race, 1985.

age 15. Provisional data for the first six months of 1987 reveal more than 9,000 cases of mumps reported.[6,8]

• In 1985, there were more than 3,500 cases of pertussis reported to the CDC. Of the 1,500 cases among children ages seven months through six years, 70% were attributable to inadequate immunization levels; one-third of these children had received no dose of the DTP vaccine at all.[7]

• In 1986, 4,195 cases of pertussis were reported—the highest number of reported cases since 1970. Sixty percent of these cases were among children under age five.[8]

State and Local

• Arizona, Arkansas, California, Florida, Illinois, New Jersey, New York City, South Carolina, Texas, and Wisconsin accounted for nearly 80% of measles cases in 1986. Outbreaks in Arizona, Florida, Illinois, New Jersey, and New York occurred mainly among unvaccinated preschool-age children.[5]

Table 1. Reported cases of selected diseases:
1979-86 and 1990 U.S. Objectives.

Year	Measles	Mumps	Pertussis
1979	13,597	14,225	1,623
1980	13,506	8,576	1,730
1981	3,124	4,941	1,248
1982	1,714	5,270	1,895
1983	1,497	3,355	2,463
1984	2,587	3,021	2,276
1985	2,822	2,982	3,589
1986	6,282	7,790	4,195
1990 Objective	500	1,000	1,000

Sources: NCHS 1986; CDC 1987d.

• In 1985, the incidence rate of mumps in states that do not require proof of immunity for school entry was twice that of states with a comprehensive K–12 mumps immunity school law.[6]

• Illinois and Tennessee accounted for one-half of the mumps cases reported in 1986.[6]

• States' immunization programs clearly have felt the effects of federal budget cuts. One Illinois county health department discontinued distribution of free vaccine to local physicians for poor children; North Carolina cut back its school record survey and measles surveillance; and in California, vaccine purchases were reduced by 10.6% in 1981, and federal funds for disease surveillance, outbreak containment, and assessment of immunization levels were cut 75%.[14]

Risk Factors

In the United States, survey data indicate that nonwhite children and children whose families are of low socioeconomic status are at increased risk of being unimmunized. In addition, children living in inner cities have consistently lower immunization rates than children living in other parts of metropolitan areas.

U.S. Objectives for Childhood Immunization Levels

The U.S. Department of Health and Human Services set forth the following objectives for increasing immunization rates among children:

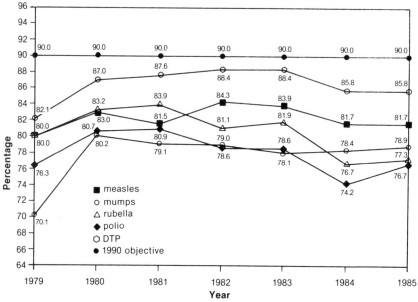

Source: National Center for Health Statistics, 1986.

Figure 4. Percentage of fully immunized two-year-olds, 1979–85 and U.S. 1990 Objective.

- By 1990, at least 90% of all children should have completed their basic immunization series by age two (measles, mumps, rubella, polio, diphtheria, pertussis, and tetanus).
- By 1990, at least 95% of children attending licensed day care facilities and kindergarten through 12th grade should be fully immunized.[19]

In 1980, more than three-fourths of two-year-olds had received vaccinations for each of the diseases specified in the first objective. However, immunization levels for 1985 were below 1980 levels for each disease. If current trends continue, the objective for two-year-olds will not be met (Figure 4).[18]

In contrast, the United States has almost achieved (or probably will soon achieve) the second objective. In the school year 1986–87, immunization levels for measles and rubella reached or exceeded the objective. Immunization levels for mumps, polio, and DTP reached or exceeded 95% for all school and day care center groups with the following exceptions: immunization rates for mumps in grades K through 12 (93%) and for polio (92%) and DTP (92%) in Head Start centers (Table 2).

The U.S. Department of Health and Human Services also established objectives for reducing vaccine-preventable diseases within the entire population:

Table 2. Percentage of children immunized by assessment instrument: school year 1986–87.

Instrument	Measles	Mumps	Rubella	Polio	DTP
Licensed Day Care Center Assessment	95	95	95	94	95
School Enterer Assessment	97	97	97	97	97
Head Start Center Assessment	95	95	95	92	92
K–12 Assessment	98	93	98	98	98

Source: CDC, 1987.

- By 1990, reported measles incidence should be reduced to fewer than 500 cases per year; mumps incidence should be reduced to fewer than 1,000 cases per year; rubella incidence should be reduced to fewer than 1,000 cases per year; congenital rubella syndrome should be reduced to fewer than 10 cases per year; diphtheria incidence should be reduced to fewer than 50 cases per year; pertussis incidence should be reduced to fewer than 1,000 cases per year; tetanus incidence should be reduced to fewer than 50 cases per year; and polio incidence should be fewer than 10 cases per year.[19]

With significant increases in reported cases of measles, mumps, and pertussis in 1986, it is unlikely that the United States will meet the objectives established for these three diseases (Table 1). The objectives for the other diseases have been or will be met.

Data Sources

State and Local

The health department of a city, county, or state is often able to provide data on immunization status at school entry (five- to six-year-olds). Depending on state requirements, a health department may also have data on immunization status for grades K through 12; certified day care facilities; and Early and Periodic Screening, Diagnosis and Treatment (EPSDT) populations. Immunization information by state and federal region is also available from the Project Head Start annual summary, the *Performance*

Indicator Report, for the three- to five-year-olds participating in the program.

National

The CDC coordinates several ongoing surveillance programs. First, the CDC gathers data on the immunization status of five- to six-year-olds through the School Entry Immunization Survey, a collection system based on annual school district reports to state and local immunization programs. The school entry data are available annually in the fact sheet *Results of School Enterer Assessments.*

Data on children through age 19 are available through 1985 from the U.S. Immunization Survey (USIS), a household survey conducted by the Census Bureau for CDC. This report provides immunization data by race (white vs. nonwhite) and age (individual years and the following age groups: younger than 1, 1–4, 5–6, 5–9, 5–14, 5–17, 10–14, 0–19, 1–19, and 15–19).

Finally, the CDC's Licensed Day Care Facilities Immunization Survey provides data on the immunization status of two-year-olds in selected day care settings. National data from this survey are considered less reliable than school entry or USIS statistics because data collection efforts vary considerably from state to state.

National data on immunization status are also available on Project Head Start and through the K–12 Assessment.

Data Needs

National

Despite the successes achieved with the 1977–79 effort to increase childhood immunization levels, and despite the recent lowering of immunization levels and increasing number of cases of debilitating diseases, surveillance of immunization status in the United States has been virtually eliminated. The results of the USIS have not been published since 1979; in 1985, the survey was discontinued altogether. Other available surveys are less comprehensive. As a result, no nationwide immunization statistics were collected by the federal government for 1986 or 1987.[13]

References

1. Banta H. Testimony before the Energy and Commerce Subcommittee on Health and the Environment, U.S. House of Representatives hearing on the effects of cuts in the Childhood Immunization Program, 4 Feb 1982. Washington, DC.

2. Centers for Disease Control. Recommendations of the Immunization Practices Advisory Committee. MMWR 1983;32(14 Jan):1–17. [Revised in 1986. See MMWR 35(19 Sep):577–9.]

3. Centers for Disease Control. Elimination of rubella and congenital rubella syndrome—United States. MMWR 1985;34(8 Feb):65–6.

4. Centers for Disease Control. Tables from the U.S. Immunization Survey, 1985. Unpublished data. Atlanta: Department of Health and Human Services, 1986.

5. Centers for Disease Control. Measles—United States, 1986. MMWR 1987;36(29 May):301–5.

6. Centers for Disease Control. Mumps—United States, 1985–1986. MMWR 1987;36(20 Mar):151–5.

7. Centers for Disease Control. Pertussis surveillance—United States, 1984 and 1985. MMWR 1987;36(27 Mar):168–71.

8. Centers for Disease Control. Summary of notifiable diseases—United States, 1986. MMWR 1987;35(25 Sep):1–48.

9. Centers for Disease Control. Tables from the Head Start Performance Indicator Report (PIR) System, 1986/87. Atlanta: Department of Health and Human Services, 1987.

10. Centers for Disease Control. Tables from the K–12 Assessment, 1986/87. Unpublished data. Atlanta: Department of Health and Human Services, 1987.

11. Centers for Disease Control. Tables from the Licensed Day Care Assessment, 1986/87. Unpublished data. Atlanta: Department of Health and Human Services, 1987.

12. Centers for Disease Control. Tables from the School Entry Assessment, 1986/87. Unpublished data. Atlanta: Department of Health and Human Services, 1987.

13. Children's Defense Fund. Who is watching our children's health?: the immunization status of American children. Washington, DC: Children's Defense Fund, 1987.

14. Glenn K. Immunization: victim of its own success? Washington Report on Medicine and Health 1982;36(20: Insert).

15. Katz S. Testimony before the Energy and Commerce Subcommittee on Health and the Environment, U.S. House of Representatives hearing on the effect of cuts in the Childhood Immunization Program, 4 Feb 1982. Washington, DC.

16. Koplan J, Schoenbaum S, Weinstein M, Fraser D. Pertussis vaccine—an analysis of benefits, risks and costs. N Engl J Med 1979;301:906–11.

17. Mausner J, Bahn A. Epidemiologic aspects of infectious disease. In: Epidemiology—an introductory text. Philadelphia: W.B. Saunders, 1974.

18. National Center for Health Statistics. Health—United States and prevention profile, 1986. DHHS Pub. No. (PHS)87–32. Washington, DC: NCHS, 1986.

19. Public Health Service. Promoting health/preventing disease: objectives for the nation. DHHS Pub. No. (OM)81–0007. Washington, DC: PHS, 1980.

20. Rappuoli R, Perugini M, Falsen E. Molecular epidemiology of the 1984–86 outbreak of diphtheria in Sweden. N Engl J Med 1988;318(1):12–4

21. Weisbrod B, Huston J. Benefits and costs of human vaccines in developed countries: an evaluative survey. Report 2 of cost-effectiveness of pharmaceuticals. Washington, DC: Pharmaceutical Manufacturers' Association, 1983.

22. White C, Koplan J, Orenstein W. Benefits, risks and costs of immunization for measles, mumps and rubella. Am J Public Health 1985;75(7):739–44.

Population-Based Growth Stunting

Definition

Population-based growth stunting is defined as a failure to achieve for a given age group a distribution of height that conforms to standards established for a well-nourished, healthy population of children. One example of population-based growth stunting would be a population group in which 15% of the children fall below the 5th percentile on standard growth charts.

Indicator

- The percentage of children in a population group whose height-for-age falls below the 5th percentile for children of the same sex and age on standard growth charts.

Significance

Health Implications

Population-based growth stunting can indicate widespread undernutrition or chronic or recurrent infections, often with intestinal parasites. It also reflects the extent of low birth weight within a population, because children born weighing less than 2,500 g are at increased risk of growth stunting, especially during the first two years of life.[9]

Although measurements of selected populations of U.S. children have helped set the standard for height distribution, studies on some isolated populations may confirm genetic differences in growth patterns. These differences are rare. Most experience indicates that as populations of "small" people achieve improved nutrition and eradication of infection, their growth patterns conform to established norms. In the United States, black children appear to grow at a slightly faster rate than white children of comparable age and nutritional status.

Growth norms are also available for head circumference and body weight. Measurements for head circumference are not readily available, however, and weight measures show greater fluctuations in rate than height and do not carry the same implications with consistency.[7, 8, 16]

Policy and Program Implications

Population-based growth stunting reflects a community's willingness and ability to provide needy children and their families with supplemental food, financial supports, health care, and sanitation services necessary to maintain adequate growth throughout pregnancy, infancy, childhood, and adolescence.

Status and Trends

National

• Data from the Centers for Disease Control (CDC) indicate that low-income children monitored by the Pediatric Nutrition Surveillance System (PedNSS) have an increased prevalence of growth stunting compared with standard reference populations. In 1986, 10.4% of CDC surveillance children fell below the 5th percentile for height. Among infants under 12 months of age, blacks evidenced the greatest growth stunting, probably reflecting the high incidence of preterm and small-for-gestational-age babies among blacks. For children one through four years of age, Asian and Pacific Islanders and Southeast Asian refugees consistently had the greatest prevalence of growth stunting, with 16.8% of one-year-olds and 18.2% of two- through four-year-olds falling below the 5th percentile for height-for-age.[5, 6]

• Over a five-year period (1979–83), 24.1% of Asian, 9.3% of Hispanic, 8.5% of white, 8.1% of Native American, and 7.5% of black children monitored by CDC fell below the 5th percentile for growth. The prevalence of growth stunting among children monitored by CDC declined slightly from 9.5% in 1976 to approximately 8.4% in 1983.[4, 21]

• Data from 1986 show 10.4% of the monitored children fell below the 5th percentile for height-for-age. These data are not comparable to earlier data, however, because new CDC editing criteria established in 1984 allow for the inclusion of more LBW (i.e., growth-stunted) babies.[6]

• Data from the second National Health and Nutrition Examination Survey (NHANES II, 1976–80) indicate that children living in poverty are at greatly increased risk of growth stunting, compared with their nonpoor peers and the standard U.S. reference population. Children aged 2 through 5 evidence the greatest disparities by poverty status, with low-income boys twice as likely as their nonpoor peers to fall below the 5th percentile for height-for-age (11.1% vs. 5.3%). Among girls ages 2 through 5, stunting is nearly three times as prevalent among low-income children as among children from higher income families (14.7% vs. 5.3%). Children aged 6 through 11 and 12 through 17 display similar disparities, with poor children 1.7 to 2.7 times as likely as nonpoor peers to be short for their age and sex.[11]

• The data from NHANES II also indicate that among rural children in the United States those from low-income families are three times more likely than nonpoor children to fall below the 5th percentile for height-for-age (7.3% vs. 2.4%). Among rural white children, 6.7% from poor families and 2.5% from nonpoor families are growth stunted; among rural nonwhite children, 8.8% from low-income families and 0.0% from higher income families fall below the 5th percentile for height-for-age.[20]

• Both the Health Examination Survey (1963–65) and the Ten-State Nutrition Survey (TSNS) (1968–70) found that children from low-income families were consistently shorter than children from higher income families. Data from the TSNS indicated that among two-year-old males from low-income families, 42% of white and 46% of black children fell below the 15th percentile for height. Similar growth retardation was noted among low-income girls, with 46% of white and 37% of black two-year-olds falling below the 15th percentile. (The TSNS did not report the percentage of children below the 5th percentile.)[10]

State and Local

Recent state and local surveillance data indicate that excessive growth stunting continues among low-income children. The Massachusetts Department of Public Health, for example, reports that 9.8% of preschoolers from low-income families throughout the commonwealth evidenced growth stunting—twice the expected rate. In Boston, 14.4% of inner-city children admitted to the Boston City Hospital emergency room fell below the 5th percentile for height—nearly three times the expected rate.[2, 13]

• Poor children in Utah experienced a remarkable rate of growth stunting. In 1986 the Utah Department of Health reported that 33% of children from low-income families (below 185% of poverty guidelines) fell below the 5th percentile for height, more than six times the predicted rate, based on national norms.[22]

• In Ramsey County, MN (St. Paul), low-income Southeast Asian children under age seven have been found to be at greatly increased risk of growth stunting compared with the standard U.S. reference population. Researchers from the University of Minnesota report that 31% of Southeast Asian youngsters studied fell below the 5th percentile for height-for-age—more than six times the expected rate. Growth stunting was more common among foreign-born children than among those born in the United States, with 40% versus 27%, respectively, falling below the 5th percentile.[3]

• The head of Chicago's Cook County Hospital emergency room found that over 30% of inner-city two-year-olds admitted to the emergency room fell under the 10th percentile for at least one growth measure.[12]

• In southern New Jersey, among low-income children aged 5 through 12, 11% of males and 10% of females were found to fall below the 5th percentile for height. Among low-income Hispanic children, 11% of males and nearly 16% of females fell below the 5th percentile for height.[19]

Risk Factors

Height is positively correlated with family income and educational status of parents. As income and educational status decrease, children tend to be shorter. National surveys indicate a small but consistent regional correlation with height: Children from the South and West tend to be smaller than peers from the Northeast and Midwest.[1, 10]

U.S. Objectives for Reduction of Growth Stunting

In 1980, the U.S. Department of Health and Human Services set the following objective for eliminating growth retardation among infants and children in this country:

• By 1990, growth retardation of infants and children caused by inadequate diets should have been eliminated in the United States as a public health problem.[17] [In 1972–73, an estimated 10% to 15% of infants and children among migratory workers and certain poor rural populations suffered growth retardation due to diet inadequacies.][17]

Data Sources

State and Local

The nutrition division of each state's health department should know the extent to which data on growth stunting are available. Some states conduct their own nutrition surveys based on a random sample of the population or on selected high-risk populations. States participating in CDC's Pediatric Nutrition Surveillance System may be able to provide data from "samples of convenience" on high-risk populations.

On the local level, the city or county health department (division of nutrition or maternal and child health) may be able to provide data, as may the local WIC (Special Supplemental Food Program for Women, Infants, and Children), Early Periodic Screening, Diagnosis, and Treatment

(EPSDT), and Head Start programs. Agencies participating in the PedNSS should have quarterly and annual printouts analyzing growth stunting among clients by age, sex, and ethnic group. Even if they are not part of the national system, some of these agencies may compile data as part of their own program reporting requirements. Although data from these programs cannot be used to generalize to an entire city or county population, they may be useful for looking at trends among selected populations.

A final source of local data may be pediatrics departments of local hospitals. In recent years, local hospitals in large cities (e.g., New York City, Boston, and Chicago) have conducted special nutritional studies of pediatric patients in emergency rooms.

National

Current national data on growth stunting are available from NCHS, CDC, and the Joint Nutrition Monitoring Evaluation Committee (JNMEC) of the U.S. Department of Health and Human Services and U.S. Department of Agriculture.

Nutrition Monitoring in the United States, first published by the JNMEC in 1986, provides a wealth of information on the nutritional status of the U.S. population, including population-based data on growth stunting among children aged 2 through 17 by age, sex, race, and poverty status (based on NHANES II data, 1976–80). The report also includes 1976–84 trend data on growth stunting among selected low-income children, by age, year, and race or ethnicity for children through age five (based on PedNSS data).[11] The JNMEC report is scheduled for publication every three years, with the next report to be issued in 1989.

The NCHS publication Vital and Health Statistics, Series 11 serves as a standard reference giving U.S. mean values and selected percentile distributions for height by age, sex, and race. The most recent Series 11 report is based on NHANES II data.[14] A Series 11 report based on data for Hispanic populations in the United States is scheduled for publication in 1989.

Additional data on growth stunting among Hispanics are available on public-use data tapes from the Hispanic Health and Nutrition Survey conducted by NCHS. Data collection for the Hispanic HANES was completed in 1984, and data tapes were first made available in 1986.

NCHS developed the standard growth chart for children in the United States based on composite data from a series of national surveys. Single copies are available from the NCHS and multiple copies from Ross Laboratories.

Extensive data on selected high-risk pediatric populations in the United States are published in *Nutrition Surveillance,* a periodic report from the PedNSS of CDC. The CDC surveillance system currently receives reports from 36 state health departments, the District of Columbia, and Puerto Rico. These reports are based primarily on data from local WIC, EPSDT, Head Start, and Maternal and Child Health programs. *Nutrition Surveillance* reports on the percentage of children (in participating programs) who fall below the 5th percentile for the standard U.S. reference population. Data are provided by age (under 3 months, 3–5 months, 6–11 months, 12–23 months, 2–5 years, and 6–9 years) and ethnic origin (white, black, Hispanic, Native American, and Asian). Five-year trend data are also available. The most recent *Nutrition Surveillance* dates from 1985 and covers 1983 data.[4]

More limited, but more timely reports from the PedNSS are published periodically in selected issues of *Morbidity and Mortality Weekly Report.* On a quarterly and annual basis, CDC also compiles data from participating states, including data on growth stunting; however, these tables are not published or as widely distributed as *Nutrition Surveillance.*

Older, but still useful background data on growth stunting are available from the first two major national nutritional surveys, both conducted in 1968 through 1970: the TSNS, which focused on low-income populations in 10 states plus New York City, and the Preschool Nutrition Survey (PNS), which looked at a random sample of U.S. children aged one to five. Reports from the TSNS are available from the Nutrition Division of the CDC. Data from the PNS are available as a supplement to *Pediatrics,* published by the American Academy of Pediatrics.[15]

Data Needs

National

Significant gaps remain in our national data system to monitor growth stunting among U.S. children. The NHANES provides population-based data, but these data are limited by infrequent collection and reporting cycles. Data collection for NHANES III began in September 1988 and will continue over a six-year period. Midpoint data covering the first three years will first be available on public-use data tapes in 1992, with publication scheduled for 1993. With 10- to 12-year intervals between studies, NHANES cannot possibly maintain a timely record of the nutritional status of the nation's children.

PedNSS data from CDC are limited because they are based on a sample of convenience, rather than a random or representative sample of the population. Thus, the CDC data do not necessarily reflect the nutritional status of all low-income children in the United States, but rather the status of children participating in certain programs in certain states. For a detailed description of the surveillance system's limitations and uses, see the CDC paper "Surveillance of Nutritional Status in the United States."[18] Reporting of annual data in *Nutrition Surveillance* has been delayed for several years, with the most recent publication covering 1983 data. It is anticipated that the report covering 1984 data will be published in 1989. In part, this delay has allowed CDC to make composite and individual state data available to participating states on a quarterly and annual basis; however, these data are not published nor are they as widely distributed as *Nutrition Surveillance*. Resumed publication of *Nutrition Surveillance* should make CDC's valuable data and analysis more accessible to a wider range of users.

References

1. American Academy of Pediatrics. The Ten-State Nutrition Survey: a pediatric perspective. AAP Newsletter Supplement, Jan 1973.

2. Brown J. Testimony before the Agriculture Subcommittee on Nutrition, U.S. Senate, 6 Apr 1983. Harvard School of Public Health. Washington, DC.

3. Brown J, Serdula M, Cairns K, Godes J, Jacobs D, Elmer P. Ethnic group differences in nutritional status of young children from low-income areas of an urban county. Am J Clin Nutr 1986;44(6):938–44.

4. Centers for Disease Control. Nutrition surveillance: annual summary 1983. DHHS Pub. No. (CDC)85–8295. Washington, DC: CDC, 1985.

5. Centers for Disease Control. Nutritional status of minority children—United States, 1986. MMWR 1987;36(23):366–9.

6. Centers for Disease Control. Table 10—pediatric nutrition surveillance: statewide summary of indicators by age and ethnic groups, reporting period 01/01/86–12/31/86. Unpublished table (26 Jun). Sequence No. 017869. Atlanta: 1987.

7. Christakis G, ed. Nutritional assessment in health programs. Am J Public Health, Supplement 1973;63(Nov):38–52.

8. Garn S, Clark D, Trowbridge F. Tendency toward greater stature in American black children. Am J Dis Child 1973;126(Aug):164–6.

9. Gayle H, Dibley M, Marks J, Trowbridge F. Malnutrition in the first two years of life: the contribution of low birth weight to population estimates in the United States. Am J Dis Child 1987;141(May):531–4.

10. Health Services Administration. The nutritional surveys. In: Health status of children: a review of surveys 1963–1972. DHEW Pub. No. (HSA)78–5744. Washington, DC: HSA, 1978.

11. Joint Nutrition Monitoring Evaluation Committee. Nutrition monitoring in the United States: a progress report from the Joint Nutrition Monitoring Evaluation Committee. DHHS Pub. No. 86–1255. Washington, DC: U.S. Department of Health and Human Services and U.S. Department of Agriculture, 1986.

12. Lattimer A. Testimony before the Subcommittee on Domestic Marketing, Consumer Relations and Nutrition, Committee on Agriculture, U.S. House of Representatives, 20 Oct 1983. Division of Ambulatory Pediatrics, Cook County Hospital. Washington, DC.

13. Massachusetts Department of Public Health. The 1983 Massachusetts Nutrition Survey. Boston: Massachusetts Department of Public Health, 1983.

14. Najjar M, Rowland M. Anthropometric reference data and prevalance of overweight: United States, 1976–80. Vital and Health Statistics, Series 11, No. 238. DHHS Pub. No. (PHS)87–1688. Washington, DC: PHS, 1987.

15. Owen G, Kram K, Garry P, Lowe J, Lubin A. A study of nutritional status of preschool children in the United States, 1968–1970. Pediatrics, Supplement Part II 1974;53(4):597–646.

16. Owen G, Lubin A. Anthropometric differences between black and white preschool children. Am J Dis Child 1973;126(Aug):168–9.

17. Public Health Service. Promoting health/preventing disease: objectives for the nation. DHHS Pub. No. (OM)81–0007. Washington, DC: PHS, 1980.

18. Robbins G. Surveillance of nutritional status in the United States. Mimeographed paper. Atlanta: Centers for Disease Control, 1980.

19. Scholl T, Karp R, Theophano J, Decker E. Ethnic differences in growth and nutritional status: a study of poor schoolchildren in southern New Jersey. Pub Health Rep 1987;102(May–Jun):278–83.

20. Shotland J. Rising poverty, declining health: the nutritional status of the rural poor. Washington, DC: Public Voice for Food and Health Policy, 1986.

21. Trowbridge F. Prevalence of growth stunting and obesity: Pediatric Nutrition Surveillance System, 1982. MMWR Surveillance Summaries 1983;32(4SS):23SSS–26SS.

22. Utah Department of Health. Summary of results of Nutrition Monitoring Project. Fact Sheet (15 Apr). Salt Lake City: Family Health Services Division, 1986.

Elevated Blood Lead Levels

Definition

An elevated blood lead level is defined as a level of lead in the blood high enough to require medical evaluation for the possibility of adverse mental, behavioral, physical, or biochemical effects.

Lead plays no known useful function in body chemistry. Although recent expert opinion suggests that any blood lead level may be adverse, the CDC has defined elevated blood lead as 25 μg or more of lead per tenth of a litre of blood (≥25 μg/dl), and the CDC recommends that children with this level of blood lead be referred for further observation and treatment. This standard was revised downward by CDC in 1985 from the previous standard of 30 μg of lead per tenth of a litre of blood.[5, 11] It is anticipated that the standard may be lowered again in the near future.[1]

Indicator

- The number of children within a defined population found to have blood lead levels of 25 μg or more per tenth of a litre of blood (≥25 μg/dl).

Significance

Health Implications

At very high doses, many organs and systems are affected by lead, including the kidney, liver, gastrointestinal tract, myocardium, immune system, blood, reproductive system (in both males and females), and central and peripheral nervous systems.[24] As a result, children with high blood lead levels may experience severe anemia, sensorimotor deficits, mental retardation, blindness, convulsions, coma, and death.[18, 22]

There is growing evidence that even at slightly elevated levels, lead exposure can produce verbal, perceptual, motor, and behavioral disabilities in children, including hearing impairment, irritability, delayed physical and neurobehavioral development, inattentiveness, inability to follow instructions, and lowered test scores for reading, spelling, and IQ.[14, 17, 20, 25, 28, 31, 32]

Exposure of the fetus to lead, even at relatively low levels, as measured from umbilical cord blood, has been associated with minor anomalies, neurobehavioral disabilities, shortened gestation, low birth weight, and growth deficits after birth.[3, 14, 21, 22, 24, 26]

Because lead can be stored in the bones, the blood lead level is an imperfect indication of the total amount of lead in the body. In times of acute illness, such as diarrhea, large amounts of lead stored in the bones may move into the blood and cause symptoms of acute lead poisoning.

Policy and Program Implications

The number of children within a defined population found to have elevated blood lead levels reflects the extent of the community's effort to regularly screen and treat high-risk populations and to reduce environmental sources of lead (e.g., lead-based paint found in old, deteriorating housing; lead plumbing in old buildings and lead soldering in new or renovated buildings; combustion of leaded gasoline, particularly in inner-city areas with heavy traffic; urban house dust; use of automobile battery casing for fuel; dietary sources, including food from cans sealed with lead soldering; exposure to certain industrial sites; and lead-containing folk remedies used by some immigrant populations).

Cost-Effectiveness of Lead Abatement and Screening Efforts

The Environmental Protection Agency (EPA) calculates that the removal of lead from gasoline can produce substantial savings resulting from improved health of both children and adults. Agency researchers project that a 90% phasedown of lead in gasoline from 1985 to 1992 would cost refineries $2.5 billion, while yielding $29.5 billion in savings related to the health of children and adults. EPA conservatively estimates cost savings specifically to children at $2.5 billion. Cost savings for adults are far greater than for children because the primary health effects for adults relate to high blood pressure and associated heart attacks and other cardiovascular disease risks, which require intensive care services in hospitals. These estimates are based on blood lead levels of 25 $\mu g/dl$ or greater and do not include a calculation of reduction in productive ability due to mental deficits related to elevated lead levels.[30, 33]

A second cost-benefit analysis conducted by the EPA concludes that a reduction of lead in drinking water would also result in substantial benefits related to the health of children. Estimates for the sample year 1988 show that a reduction in exposure to lead in drinking water from the current EPA drinking water standard of 50 $\mu g/l$ (or parts per billion) to the proposed standard of 20 $\mu g/l$ would cost about $230 million annually. Estimates of the annual benefits related to children's health range from $109 to $296 million, depending on the method used to estimate the costs of cognitive damage. An estimate of nonmonetary benefits for children shows the following annual reductions in the numbers of children at risk: 29,000 fewer children requiring medical treatment; 241,000 fewer children losing 1 to 5 IQ points; 29,000 fewer children requiring compensatory education; 82,000 fewer children at risk of growth stunting; and 82,400 fewer children at increased risk of hematological effects.[16]

Lead screening has been determined to be highly cost-effective. According to a June 1982 report in the *New England Journal of Medicine,* in areas where the prevalence of lead toxicity is 7% or more, lead screening averts morbidity and results in net dollar savings.[4] If calculations take into account quality of life and other noneconomic benefits, lead-screening programs are highly cost-effective even at prevalence rates as low as 1% to 2%.[15]

Status and Trends

National

• The Agency for Toxic Substances and Disease Registry (ATSDR) estimates that between 3 and 4 million children in the United States under age six have blood lead levels above 15 μg/dl, a level associated with the onset of early detectable adverse effects. In metropolitan areas, an estimated 17% of youngsters under age six have blood lead levels over 15 μg/dl.[21]

• In U.S. metropolitan areas, an estimated 5.2% of children under age six—some 715,000 youngsters—have blood lead levels greater than 20 μg/dl, and 1.4% of youngsters under age six—nearly 200,000 children—have blood lead levels greater than the current CDC standard of 25 μg/dl.[12, 22]

• Data from the second National Health and Nutrition Examination Survey (NHANES II, 1976–80) indicate that among U.S. children six months through five years old, black children are six times as likely as white children to have blood lead levels of 30 μg/dl or greater. Young children from very poor families are nine times more likely to have blood lead levels of 30 μg/dl or greater than are children from families with higher incomes, and children living in central cities of large urban areas are more than five times as likely as rural children to have blood lead levels at or above 30 μg/dl.[2]

• Although poor, inner-city children have an increased prevalence of lead toxicity, no social, economic, or racial group is exempt from lead exposure and its effects. More affluent, non-inner-city children make up a very large portion of the population and add substantially to the total number of U.S. children with elevated blood lead levels.[21]

• Trend data from NHANES II (1976–80) indicate that mean blood lead levels have decreased among U.S. children. This decline has been closely correlated with reductions in the lead content of gasoline. Although this trend is encouraging, a great deal of evidence amassed since 1980 shows that blood lead levels previously thought to be safe can result in adverse effects. The net result is that the total number of children considered at risk of adverse effects resulting from lead exposure has increased in recent years.[2, 12]

• Since the early 1970s, when lead-screening programs were first established, they have undergone changes in administration, organization, funding levels, and definitions of toxicity, all of which make it difficult to use program data to monitor trends over time. Nevertheless, ATSDR has reviewed program data available to date and has concluded that they show trends consistent with trends noted in NHANES II data. Specifically, from 1973 onward there has been a moderate decline in the proportion of children with confirmed lead toxicity, presumably reflecting decreases in environmental lead contamination. Further, available data indicate that as CDC revises risk classifications in recognition of the fact that relatively low levels of lead exposure result in adverse effects, the proportion of children considered at risk will increase.[22]

• An ATSDR analysis of the sources of lead exposure in the United States indicates that leaded paint "has been and remains a major source of childhood lead exposure and intoxication" and that lead in dust and soil runs close to leaded paint as a persistent and widespread source of exposure. Although drinking water has recently been recognized as a significant source of lead, leaded gasoline and lead in food have declined in importance in the United States.[22]

• An estimated 13.6 million U.S. children under age seven are potentially exposed to lead-based paint in concentrations high enough to cause adverse effects. Between 5.9 and 11.7 million U.S. children are exposed to dangerously high levels of lead in soil and dust.[22]

• An estimated 6.6 million children under age 14 are exposed to lead in tap water (from either old pipes or lead soldering in new plumbing), and an estimated 241,000 children under age six suffer blood lead levels greater than 15 $\mu g/dl$ as a result of drinking contaminated water. Many experts believe that current lead levels in drinking water are too high. In 1985, the EPA proposed cutting the acceptable limit by more than half, from 50 to 20 μg of lead per litre of water. In August 1988, EPA proposed a further reduction to 5 μg/l in the water distribution system and average levels of 10 μg/l at home taps. No final action has been taken to date, and evidence continues to mount that even the most recent proposal does not adequately protect public health.[21, 34, 36]

State and Local

• Because state and local data on lead exposure among children are almost exclusively derived from lead-screening programs, the data reflect lead exposure or toxicity rates among selected high-risk populations of children rather than population-based prevalence rates. Additionally, screening results are not necessarily comparable from one program to the next because reporting requirements vary with locality. Despite these limitations, ATSDR reviewed findings from some 40 to 45 existing programs and reports that in 1985, the proportion of children found to have lead toxicity ranged from 0.3% in five programs to 11.0% in the city of St. Louis, MO. The programs reporting the highest rates of lead toxicity were St. Louis (11.0%); Augusta and Savannah, GA (9.0%); Harrisburg, PA (4.9%); Washington, DC (3.5%); and Merrimac Valley, MA (3.5%). In most programs fewer than 2.0% of screened children had confirmed lead toxicity.[22]

• ATSDR researchers note that lead toxicity rates based on state and local screening data generally are lower than prevalence rates projected from NHANES II data. Reasons cited for this disparity include high false negative rates associated with the screening test most lead programs use and the screening of clinic populations rather than intensive house-to-house testing in high-risk areas. ATSDR scientists also note that a high reported rate of toxicity may not necessarily mean that the community has an "exceptional lead exposure situation," but rather may mean that the lead program is doing an exceptionally thorough job of screening high-risk populations.[22]

• Pennsylvania is one state that has used population-based data to estimate the number of children with lead toxicity. Using NHANES II and U.S. Census data to project the extent of lead toxicity among all children in the state, Pennsylvania health officials estimated that more than 19,000 children under age six had lead levels considered unsafe under CDC guidelines. In high-risk areas of the state, prevalence rates exceeded 18%, and in no county did prevalence fall below 1%. It should be noted that these estimates were based on CDC's pre-1985 standard of 30 μg/dl.[35]

- New York State, which is considered to have the largest screening program in the nation, reports that in 1985, more than 250,000 children were screened for lead. The confirmed lead poisoning case rate for screened children in New York City was 5.9% (11,600 children). For communities with screening programs in the remainder of the state, the lead poisoning case rate among screened children was 4.0% (more than 2,100 children).[13]

- Massachusetts has the highest statewide screening penetration in the nation—40% in 1986. (In high-risk urban areas, screening penetration reached 72%.) The statewide incidence of lead poisoning among screened children (under age six) was 0.7% in 1986, and no community had an incidence rate higher than 2.0% among screened children. The Massachusetts lead poisoning prevention program is one of the bright lights among efforts to address the adverse effects of lead among children. Between 1985 and 1986, the number of new cases of lead poisoning in the state declined 40%, and the number of severely poisoned children dropped 30%. Still, more than 1,000 Massachusetts children suffered from lead poisoning in 1986, a number state officials consider "unacceptably high for a preventable disease."[23]

Risk Factors

Many characteristics affect an individual's vulnerability to lead. These include genetic variations in susceptibility, nutritional status, behavior, and age.[24] Young children under age six are particularly vulnerable to the effects of lead. In some instances, an entire population can be exposed, but only the children will show dangerously high blood lead levels.

Although elevated lead levels are found in children of all races and socioeconomic standing, black, poor, and inner-city children are at greatest risk for elevated blood lead levels. Excess lead exposure is associated with a variety of demographic risk factors, such as large family size, number of preschool children in the family (risk increases as number of preschoolers increases), deteriorated housing, low socioeconomic status, marital separation of parents, unemployment of parents, absence of parents, lack of day care facilities, and poor maternal prenatal nutrition.[19,24] In addition, certain immigrant populations (Mexican-Hispanic, Hmong, and Asian Indian) are at increased risk because of lead-containing folk remedies.[6,8,10]

U.S. Objective for Reducing Adverse Effects of Lead

In 1980, the Department of Health and Human Services developed the following outcome objective for reducing adverse effects of lead among our nation's children:

- By 1990, 80% of communities should experience a prevalence rate of lead toxicity of less than 500/100,000 among children age 0–5, especially from ages 0–1.[29] [In 1980, the estimated prevalence of lead toxicity nationally exceeded 1,000/100,000.][29]

Data Sources

State and Local

As noted earlier in the text, state and local data on lead exposure among children are almost exclusively derived from lead-screening programs. Often, the maternal and child health division or family health division within a state health agency is a source of both local and composite state data from lead programs. For fiscal year 1984, approximately half of the state health agencies could provide composite data on the number of children screened and the proportion requiring further diagnostic evaluation.

The city or county health department (maternal and child health or environmental health division) is the agency most likely to have local lead program data. In communities that do not have lead programs, some data may be available from hospitals providing lead screening and treatment to pediatric patients.

Three additional sources provide screening and evaluation data from various state and local programs: the ATSDR report to Congress, *The Nature and Extent of Lead Poisoning in Children in the United States*[22] (the most current and most comprehensive source); the Public Health Foundation's annual report *Public Health Agencies, Vol. 3, Services for Mothers and Children*[27] (data from FY 1982 forward); and the CDC publication *Morbidity and Mortality Weekly Report (MMWR)*[6-8, 10, 12] (data from 1972 to 1982). A more detailed review of these publications is in the following section, on national data sources.

National

The most current and most comprehensive source of national data is the 1988 report by the ATSDR, *The Nature and Extent of Lead Poisoning in Children in the United States: A Report to Congress.*[22] This publication provides new population-based estimates of the number of children at risk of adverse effects of lead exposure, reports on lead exposure by source, compiles state and local screening data, discusses difficulties in assessing trends and in comparing data from existing programs, analyzes data gaps and research needs, and provides recommendations on a wide set of activities to be undertaken in order to eliminate childhood lead poisoning in the United States.

There is no annual source of population-based data on lead exposure and toxicity. The first and only national population-based survey of blood lead levels completed to date is NHANES II, conducted by the National Center for Health Statistics (NCHS) from 1976 through 1980. NCHS published findings from NHANES II in *Advance Data from Vital and Health Statistics*[2] and in the *New England Journal of Medicine*.[19] Data are analyzed by age, race, sex, family income, and degree of urbanization. Some trend information is also available. NHANES II data are the basis of newer population-based estimates reported by the ATSDR in 1988.

Data on blood lead levels among Hispanic populations in the United States were collected as part of the Hispanic Health and Nutrition Examination Survey, which was completed in December 1984. The survey focused on Mexican-Americans, Puerto Ricans, and Cuban-Americans. It is anticipated that Hispanic HANES data on 4- through 11-year-olds, including mean blood lead levels and percentage with elevated blood lead, will be published by 1989.

The next National Health and Nutrition Examination Survey (NHANES III) will include nationally representative data on lead exposure levels, as well as data on the extent of screening and treatment. Data collection for the survey began in September 1988 and will continue over a six-year period. It is anticipated that midpoint data, covering the first three years of the survey, will first be available on data tapes in 1992, with published data available in the following year.

Composite data from lead-screening programs throughout the country are available annually in the Public Health Foundation's report *Public Health Agencies, Vol. 3, Services for Mothers and Children*. Starting with FY 1982, the Public Health Foundation (formerly the Association of State and Territorial Health Officers) has published data voluntarily reported by state health agencies, including the estimated number of children aged one through five at risk, the number screened, and the number and percentage requiring diagnostic evaluation, receiving diagnostic evaluation, and with confirmed lead toxicity. Data from 1984 are based on reporting from 26 state health agencies.[27]

Between 1972 and 1982, the CDC published data from state and local lead programs receiving federal funding. Information on the number of children screened, requiring pediatric care, and receiving care was published annually and quarterly in *MMWR*.[9] When federal funds for lead screening were shifted from CDC to the Maternal and Child Health block grant, a number of programs were eliminated and reporting became voluntary. As a result, CDC had insufficient data to report accurately on trends, and publication in *MMWR* was discontinued starting with 1983 data.

Data Needs

National

There is a great need for more frequent collection, analysis, and dissemination of population-based data on lead exposure among U.S. children. Data from NHANES have proven invaluable in assessing the extent of lead toxicity nationwide; however, at best, NHANES is conducted only once every 10 years. As new evidence mounts, showing adverse effects associated with blood lead levels previously thought to be safe, the need for accurate, current population-based data becomes all the more pressing.

Data from screening and treatment programs need to be collected and assessed more systematically and comprehensively. Currently, the Public Health Foundation, the only source of annual data on activities and findings of screening programs nationwide, must rely on voluntary reporting by state health agencies. For FY 1984, only 26 states reported on the number of children screened, and only 22 reported on the percentage of screened children who had confirmed lead toxicity. In addition, data are not uniform from program to program, making it very difficult to assess trends nationwide. Mandatory reporting of data to a federal government agency using uniform reporting criteria would do much to improve the situation.

References

1. American Academy of Pediatrics. Statement on childhood lead poisoning. Pediatrics 1987;(3 Mar):457–65.

2. Annest J, Mahaffey K, Cox D, Roberts J. Blood lead levels for persons 6 months–74 years of age: United States 1976–80. advance data (12 May). Washington, DC: National Center for Health Statistics, 1982.

3. Bellinger D, Leviton A, Waternaux C, Needleman H, Rabinowitz M. Longitudinal analyses of prenatal and postnatal lead exposure and early cognitive development. N Engl J Med 1987;316(Apr):1037–43.

4. Berkwick D, Komaroff A. Cost-effectiveness of lead screening. N Engl J Med 1982;306(10 Jun):1392–8.

5. Centers for Disease Control. Preventing lead poisoning in young children: a statement by the Centers for Disease Control. Atlanta: U.S. Department of Health, Education, and Welfare, 1978.

6. Centers for Disease Control. Use of lead tetroxide as a folk remedy for gastrointestinal illness. MMWR 1981;30:456–547.

7. Centers for Disease Control. Lead poisoning from lead tetroxide used as a folk remedy—Colorado. MMWR 1982;30:647–8.

8. Centers for Disease Control. Folk remedy–associated lead poisoning in Hmong children—Minnesota. MMWR 1983;32:555–6.

9. Centers for Disease Control. Lead poisoning. MMWR – Annual Summary 1983;31(54). Public Health Service. DHHS Pub. No. (CDC)84–8241. Washington, DC.

10. Centers for Disease Control. Lead poisoning–associated death from Asian Indian folk remedies—Florida. MMWR 1984;33:638–45.

11. Centers for Disease Control. Preventing lead poisoning in young children: a statement by the Centers for Disease Control. Atlanta: U.S. Department of Health and Human Services, 1985.

12. Centers for Disease Control. Childhood lead poisoning—United States: report to the Congress by the Agency for Toxic Substances and Disease Registry. MMWR 1988;37:481–5.

13. Child and Adolescent Health Profile Project. Child and adolescent health profile: New York State 1985. Albany, NY: Welfare Research Institute, 1988.

14. Davis J, Svendsgaard D. Lead and child development. Nature 1987;329(24 Sep):297–300.

15. Division of Maternal and Child Health. Cost-effectiveness of lead screening. Memo. Oct. Washington, DC: Public Health Service, 1982.

16. Levin R. Reducing lead in drinking water: a benefit analysis. EPA Document No. 230–09–86–019. Washington, DC: U.S. Environmental Protection Agency, 1986.

17. Lin-Fu J. Vulnerability of children to lead exposure and toxicity. N Engl J Med 1973;289(Dec):1229–33, 1289–93.

18. Lin-Fu J. What price shall we pay for lead poisoning in children? Children Today 1979;8(Jan–Feb):9–13.

19. Lin-Fu J. Children and lead: new findings and concerns. N Engl J Med 1982;307(2 Sep):615–7.

20. Mahaffey K, Annest L, Roberts J, Murphy R. National estimates of blood lead levels: United States 1976–80. N Engl J Med 1982;307(2 Sep)573–9.

21. Mushak P, Crocetti A. Testimony before the Subcommittee on Health and Environment, Committee on Energy and Commerce, U.S. House of Representatives, 10 Dec 1987. University of North Carolina and New York Medical College. Washington, DC.

22. Mushak P, Crocetti A. The nature and extent of lead poisoning in children in the United States: a report to Congress. Atlanta: Agency for Toxic Substances and Disease Registry, U.S. Public Health Service, 1988.

23. National Coalition on Prevention of Mental Retardation. The Massachusetts Lead Program: moving toward Phase 2. Prevention Update 1987(Apr).

24. Needleman H, Bellinger D. The developmental consequences of childhood exposure to lead: recent studies and methodological issues. Advances in Clinical Child Psychology 1984;7:195–220.

25. Needleman H, Gunnoe C, Leviton A, Reed R, Peresie H, Maher C, Barrett P. Deficits in psychologic and classroom performance of children with elevated dentine lead levels. N Engl J Med 1979;300(29 Mar):689–95.

26. Needleman H, Rabinowitz M, Leviton A, Linn S, Schoenbaum S. The relationship between prenatal exposure to lead and congenital anomalies. JAMA 1984;251(22):2956–9.

27. Public Health Foundation. Adolescent and child health. In: Public health agencies 1984; vol 3, Services for mothers and children. Washington, DC: Public Health Foundation, 1987:11–13.

28. Public Health Service. Healthy people: the Surgeon General's report on health promotion and disease prevention, background papers. DHEW Pub. No. (PHS)79-55071A. Washington, DC: PHS, 1979.

29. Public Health Service. Promoting health/preventing disease: objectives for the nation. DHHS Pub. No. (OM)81-0007. Washington, DC: PHS, 1980.

30. Schwartz J. Private communication with authors. 21 Mar 1988. Harvard University, School of Public Health. Boston, MA.

31. Schwartz J, Angle C, Pitcher H. Relationship between childhood blood lead levels and stature. Pediatrics 1986;77(Mar):281-8.

32. Schwartz J, Otto D. Blood lead, hearing thresholds, and neurobehavioral development in children and youth. Achievers of Environmental Health 1987;42(May/June):153-60.

33. Schwartz J, Pitcher H., Levin R, Ostrow B, Nichols A. Costs and benefits of reducing lead in gasoline. EPA Document No. 230-05-85-006. Washington, DC: U.S. Environmental Protection Agency, 1985.

34. Silbergeld E. Testimony before the Subcommittee on Health and the Environment, Committee on Energy and Commerce, U.S. House of Representatives, 10 Dec 1987. Washington, DC.

35. Tucker A. Program for the Control of Childhood Lead Poisoning Within the Commonwealth of Pennsylvania, as administered under the Department of Health's Maternal and Child Health Block Grant—Program Description. Harrisburg, PA: Pennsylvania Department of Health and Pennsylvania State Data Center, 1983.

36. Waxman H. Opening statement for Hearing on Lead Contamination in Drinking Water, Subcommittee on Health and Environment, Committee on Energy and Commerce, U.S. House of Representatives, 10 Dec 1987. Washington, DC.

Non–Motor Vehicle Accident Fatalities

Definition

An accident or injury fatality is a death that results from an unanticipated and unintended event. Drowning, fires and burns, and falls are among the leading causes of accidental death among children and youths. Other major causes of non–motor vehicle accident fatalities in childhood include aspiration of food and objects, poisoning by solids or liquids, and poisoning by gas.

Indicator

- The rate of non–motor vehicle accident fatalities (deaths per 100,000 population) for the following age groups: under 1, 1–4, 5–9, 10–14, and 15–19.

Significance

Health Implications

> Vulnerable infants cannot perceive dangers in their environment, and even if they do primitively perceive danger, they cannot move out of harm's way. Toddlers 'toddle'; hence their predisposition to physical injury. Their natural curiosity, unbalanced by wisdom, can result in the exploration of dangerous areas and chemicals. School-age children are carefree and careless; both qualities are essential for a happy and explorative childhood but are inimical to life and limb in a hazardous environment. Teenagers are risk takers; that is a part of growing up. If they are lucky, risk taking makes for more mature adults; unlucky ones can wind up in the hospital or morgue. Such is the road to maturity, filled with natural and unnatural hazards.[6]

Nonfatal injuries account for half of all visits to hospital emergency rooms.[3] Millions of children are injured seriously enough each year to require some kind of medical treatment. Children who survive potentially fatal accidental injuries may suffer severe permanent physical or mental damage requiring extensive treatment or extended care. Possible consequences to survivors include brain damage, broken bones, spinal cord injury, injury to internal organs, extensive scarring, loss of limbs or loss of the use of limbs, and loss of vision or hearing.

Policy and Program Implications

A broad range of preventive measures can affect the rate of non–motor vehicle accident fatalities among children and youths. Preventive efforts can encompass legislative, regulatory, and educational strategies. The rate of death from non–motor vehicle accidents reflects the extent to which a society effectively regulates the safety of consumer products, implements and enforces codes to assure safe and adequate housing, provides adequate child care for working parents, maintains safe public spaces, provides poison control hotlines, assures access to services and emergency medical care when an injury does occur, promotes the use of child-proof packaging for potential poisons, and educates the public regarding accident prevention. A higher rate of accident fatalities among some subpopulations reflects disparities in income, housing, and education.

Status and Trends

• In 1985, non–motor vehicle accidents accounted for 40% of all accidental deaths during childhood. More than 6,400 U.S. children and youths under age 20 died as a result of injury in non–motor vehicle accidents.[13, 14]

• Overall, the lowest rates of death are among children ages 5 to 9. In 1985, the rate of non–motor vehicle accident fatalities for this age group was 5.5 per 100,000. The rates for other age groups were as follows: infants under age 1, 19.0; preschoolers ages 1 to 4, 12.9; adolescents ages 10 to 14, 5.9; and teens ages 15 to 19, 10.3[14] (Figure 5).

• Although rates of accidental death have been converging for white and black youths ages 15 to 19, racial disparities persist for children under age 15. In 1985, the rate of non–motor vehicle accident fatalities among black infants was twice the rate for white infants; among children ages 1 to 4, the rate for blacks was 1.6 times the rate for whites; among 5- to 9-year olds, the rate for black children was 2.2 times the rate for whites; and black adolescents ages 10 to 14 sustained fatal injuries at a rate 1.6 times the rate for white adolescents[14] (Figure 5).

• For all race and sex combinations, the highest rate of non–motor vehicle accident fatalities in childhood occurs among black infants under age one. In 1985, 33.2 out of every 100,000 black babies died as a result of non–motor vehicle accidents[14] (Figure 5).

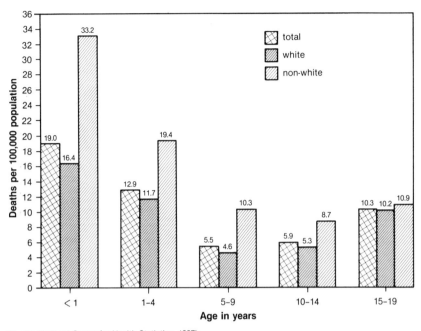

Source: National Center for Health Statistics, 1987b.

Figure 5. Rates of non–motor vehicle accident fatalities by age and race, 1985.

- Children under one year of age have more deaths from accidents than children of any other age. About half of all accidental deaths in the first year of life are among babies under five months of age; more than two-thirds are among infants younger than seven months.[11]

- For all ages during childhood, males are more likely to sustain fatal injuries than females. This pattern is true for each cause of accidental death.[14]

- In 1986, falls, drowning, and fires and burns were the leading causes of non–motor vehicle accidental deaths.[15]

- In 1985, preschoolers ages 1 to 4 accounted for nearly 47% of all people under age 20 who died as a result of fires and for one-third of all children who drowned. Among children who died from falls, 40% were ages 15 to 19.[14]

- In 1985, the number of deaths from falls (328) was relatively low for people under age 20. However, the total number of fall-related deaths may have been underreported because falls initiating or contributing to further complications may not be listed on death certificates as the cause of death.[2, 14]

• Between 1984 and 1985, there was essentially no change in the rate of deaths from falls for children ages 1 to 19, but the rate for infants under age 1 increased 50%—from 0.8 to 1.2 per 100,000. Falls accounted for 5% of all accidental deaths in this age group.[14]

• Between 1984 and 1985, the rate of deaths from drowning increased for every age group of children.[14]

• The rate of death from drowning is higher for black children than for white children at every age, with the exception of the preschool years (ages one to four), when white children drown at more than twice the rate of black children[14] (Table 3).

• Rates of fire-related deaths have been falling steadily in recent years. Nonetheless, in 1985, these rates were disproportionately higher for black children than white children. Death rates from fires and burns were also higher for males than females, and higher among one- to four-year-olds than among children in any other age group[14] (Table 3).

Risk Factors

At greatest risk of non–motor vehicle accidental injury are children and youths from low-income and poorly educated families, those who live in inadequate or deteriorating housing, and those living under unusually stressful conditions.[8, 9, 19, 20] There is also some evidence that children with a history of injury are at increased risk of subsequent accidental injury.[5, 20] Alcohol and drug abuse increase the risk of home accident fatalities among youths ages 15 to 19.[7, 16]

Table 3. Accident fatality rates (number per 100,000 population) by cause, age, and race: 1985.

Age	Drowning			Fires and Burns			Falls		
	All Races	White	Black	All Races	White	Black	All Races	White	Black
Under 1	2.3	2.3	2.8	3.0	2.1	8.1	1.2	0.9	2.3
1–4	4.1	4.4	2.0	4.3	3.2	10.9	0.6	0.4	1.2
5–9	1.5	1.2	2.8	1.8	1.2	5.1	0.2	0.1	0.3
10–14	1.6	1.1	4.4	0.9	0.7	1.9	0.3	0.3	0.2
15–19	3.0	2.7	4.8	0.7	0.6	1.2	0.7	0.8	0.2

Source: National Center for Health Statistics, 1987b.

An increased risk for accidental injury and death during early childhood reflects various aspects of physical and mental development: recognition of hazards, curiosity, the ability to perform certain tasks, and the need for supervision.[2,6] Particularly at young ages, black children are at greater risk of accidental death than white children.

Maternal age, parity, and birth order of the child may also serve as predictors of risk. Research suggests that the younger the mother, the greater the risk of accidental death during a child's first year of life. Rates of accident fatalities for children under age one year also tend to increase as the number of children in the family increases.[21] Children born to teenage mothers are at increased risk of nonfatal accidental injury during the first five years of life.[1] The risk of nonfatal injury for a preschool-age child appears to decrease if the child has an older sibling. In adolescence, however, this trend is reversed, with children having an older sibling being at increased risk of injury.[10]

Generally, boys are at greater risk than girls for accidental injury.[15] The increased risk among boys, especially as age increases, may be a function of differences in risk-taking behavior.[18]

U.S. Objective for Reducing the Rate of Non–Motor Vehicle Accident Fatalities

The U.S. Department of Health and Human Services set the following objective for reducing the rate of home accident fatalities among children. (Home accident fatalities are a subset of non–motor vehicle accident fatalities.)

- By 1990, the rate of home accident fatalities for children under age 15 should be no greater than 5.0 per 100,000 children.[17]

Between 1978 and 1984, the rate of deaths resulting from home injuries among children younger than 15 years decreased from 6.0 per 100,000 to the 1990 Objective of 5.0.[12]

Although the 1990 Objectives include goals for reducing death rates from falls, drowning, and fires and burns, these objectives are for the population as a whole, not specifically for children, and are not reported here.

Data Sources

State and Local

The registrar of vital statistics, usually located within the state or local health department, maintains accident fatality data compiled from death certificates. In some states and localities, the medical examiner's office may provide data on accident fatalities. State and local burn registries, poison control centers, and divisions within health departments (emergency medical services, maternal and child health, and environmental health) are also sources of data on specific kinds of accidental injury.

The CDC provides communities technical assistance on collecting and analyzing data through its *Injury Control Surveys.*[4] Analysis of data from the surveys provide information on the type, extent, severity, and cost of each injury and reflects the impact of interventions on mortality and morbidity for a specific subpopulation or geographic area or for the community as a whole.

Some states, such as Maryland and Massachusetts, have established a system for collecting population-based data on injury mortality and morbidity in childhood. The Public Health Foundation (formerly the Association of State and Territorial Health Officials) also maintains information on states' accident prevention programs.

National

NCHS publishes comprehensive data on non–motor vehicle accident fatalities annually in *Vital Statistics of the United States, Vol. II, Mortality.* There is approximately a three-year lag between the end of a calendar year and publication of data for that year. Based on data from state death certificates, this publication reports the total number of non–transport accident fatalities by age, race, sex, and external cause. Also, the number of non–transport accident fatalities by place is reported by age, race, and sex.

A more timely, but less comprehensive source of data is the *Advance Report of Final Mortality Statistics,* part of the NCHS Monthly Vital Statistics Report series. This report provides annual data on non–motor vehicle accident fatalities and fatality rates (listed as "all other accidents and adverse effects") by age group (under 1, 1–4, 5–14, and 15–24). For infants, accident fatalities are also stratified by race (white, black, and all other). Approximately two years after the end of a calendar year, the data for that year are available.

Under its Injury Prevention Initiative, the CDC provides information on mortality and morbidity from fires and burns, drownings, falls, and other injuries occurring in the home. Based on reports from state health departments, the data are published periodically in the *Morbidity and Mortality Weekly Report.*

Another source of data on accident fatalities is *Accident Facts,* published annually by the National Safety Council. This publication provides trend data on total accident fatalities and on fatality rates by age group (under

5, 5–14, and 15–24). It also reports the current incidence of accident fatalities for each age group by type of accident (drowning, fires and burns, falls, ingestion of food and objects, firearms, poisoning by solid or liquid, and poisoning by gas) and by percentage of fatal accidents to males. Total accidental deaths and death rates are estimated for the most recent years up to and including the year prior to the publication date.

The Consumer Product Safety Commission (CPSC) publishes information on accident fatalities associated with specific consumer products. These data are based on the National Electronic Injury Surveillance System, a nationally representative survey of emergency room injuries and fatalities associated with consumer products. The CPSC also produces a series of special Hazard Analysis Reports, which include data on deaths and injuries by age, as well as summaries of the circumstances leading up to the accident in some cases.

The National Fire Incident Reporting System, run by the National Fire Data Center of the Federal Emergency Management Agency, has been in existence since 1976. From the individual fire department involved, the system collects data on the state in which the fire occurred, sex and rate of individuals killed or injured in the fire, cause of the fire, type of building or residence, and cause of death or injury. In addition, the presence or absence of smoke detectors is noted.

The National Burn Information Exchange is a private effort run by the National Institute of Burn Medicine in Ann Arbor, MI. As of January 1980, the data base included information on nearly 47,000 burn patients treated at 125 burn care facilities. Data collected include age, sex, and race of the injured person; date and location where the injury occurred; date of hospital admission, discharge, or death; cause of the injury; and medical treatment given.

Data from selected local, state, and regional poison control centers are available from the Poisoning Surveillance and Epidemiology Branch of the Food and Drug Administration (FDA). FDA's annual *Poison Control Case Summary* reports product- or substance-specific exposures and fatalities by age of child (under five and five and older).

Data Needs

National

There is a three-year lag between the end of a calendar year and publication of final national data for that year. This relatively long lag makes it difficult to use timely data for purposes of evaluating, planning, and implementing public policies and programs.

Another limitation of vital statistics data is the lack of information on the circumstances under which injury deaths occur. Currently, there is no national data base that links the external cause of injurious death with the nature of the injury sustained and the precipitating circumstances.

In addition to the gaps in our information base, there remains a discrepancy between what is already known about the cause and prevention of accidents and the application of that knowledge. Existing national data bases must be integrated and expanded to facilitate the design and evaluation of prevention programs and to further research efforts in this area.

References

1. Alan Guttmacher Institute. Children born to teens more likely to be injured or hospitalized by age 5. Fam Plann Perspect 1983;16(Sep–Oct):238.

2. Baker S, O'Neill B, Karpf R. The injury fact book. Lexington, MA: Lexington Books, 1984.

3. Barancik J, Chatterjee B, Greene Y, Michenzi E, Fife D. Northeastern Ohio Trauma Study: I. magnitude of the problem. Am J Public Health 1983;73:746–51.

4. Centers for Disease Control. Injury Control Surveys: training resource manual. DHHS Pub. No. (CDC)83–8344. Atlanta: CDC, 1983.

5. Feldman K. Prevention of childhood accidents: recent progress. Pediatrics in Review 1980;2(3):75–81.

6. Fulginiti V. Our children are being maimed and killed. Am J Dis Child 1987;141(Dec):1255.

7. Howland J, Hingson R. Alcohol as a risk factor for injuries or death due to fires and burns: review of the literature. Public Health Reports 1987;102(Sep–Oct):475–83.

8. Locke J, Rossignol A, Boyle C, Burke J. Socioeconomic factors and burn rates in persons hospitalized for burns in Massachusetts. Public Health Reports 1986;101(Jul–Aug):389–95.

9. Maine Department of Human Services. Children's deaths in Maine. 1976–1980 Final Report. Augusta: Maine Department of Human Services, 1983.

10. Manheimer D, Dewey J, Mellinger G, Corsa L. 50,000 child-years of accidental injuries. Public Health Reports 1966;81(6):519–32.

11. Metropolitan Life Insurance Company. The risky first year of life. Statistical Bulletin 1985;(Jan–Mar):2–8.

12. National Center for Health Statistics. Health—United States and prevention profile, 1986. DHHS Pub. No. (PHS)87–32. Washington, DC: NCHS, 1986.

13. National Center for Health Statistics. Advance report of final mortality statistics, 1985. Monthly Vital Statistics Report 36(28 Aug). Supplement. DHHS Pub. No. 87–1120. Washington, DC: NCHS, 1987.

14. National Center for Health Statistics. Death from each cause by 5-year age groups, race and sex: United States, 1985. Unpublished data. Washington, DC, 1987.

15. National Safety Council. Accident facts, 1987 edition. Chicago: National Safety Council, 1987.

16. Planek T. Home accidents: a continuing problem. Accid Anal Prev 1982;14(2): 107–20.

17. Public Health Service. Promoting health/preventing disease: objectives for the nation. DHHS Pub. No. (OM)81–0007. Washington, DC: PHS, 1980.

18. Rivara F, Bergman A, LoGerfo J, Weiss N. Epidemiology of childhood injuries: II. sex differences in injury rates. Am J Dis Child 1982;136(Jun):502–6.

19. Schor E. Unintentional injuries: patterns within families. Am J Dis Child 1987;141(Dec):1280–4.

20. Walker B, Raines D. Childhood accidents in a rural community: a five-year study. J Fam Pract 1982;14(4):705–8.

21. Wicklund K, Moss S, Frost F. Effects of maternal education, age and parity on fatal infant accidents. Am J Public Health 1984;74(10):1150–2.

CHAPTER 4

Indicators of Special Importance to Adolescents and Young Adults

Births to School-Age Mothers

Indicator

- The number of births to mothers under age 15 and ages 15 to 17 per 1,000 females in each age group.

Significance

Implications for Health and Social Functioning

For a combination of physiological, social, and economic reasons, teenage childbearing is associated with a variety of negative consequences for both the mothers and their babies.

Consequences for the babies: Infants born to school-age mothers are at increased risk of being born prematurely and of dying before they reach their first birthdays; they are also more likely to be of low birth weight than are infants born to women in their 20's.[3, 24, 26] Young maternal age may be a predictor of sudden infant death, gastrointestinal problems, and accidents.[4, 22] Later in life, children born to teenage mothers are less likely than other children to adapt well to school, are likely to score lower than other children on IQ tests, are at increased risk of being educationally and emotionally compromised, and are at risk for teen pregnancy.[6, 17] Additionally, there is some evidence that children born to young mothers may be at increased risk of neglect, mental retardation, congenital defects, and other handicapping conditions.[2, 5, 21, 26]

Consequences for the mothers: Although early childbearing is associated with some adverse health consequences, these effects seem to be largely a function of the interaction of a number of economic and psychosocial variables rather than due to biologic factors.[3, 5] In studies where maternal outcome varies by age, these differences are usually in measures that are sensitive to socioeconomic factors, such as complications of toxemia and iron deficiency anemia, and not in biologically constrained outcomes of labor and delivery.[22, 41]

Beyond health consequences, school-age childbearing subverts the usual transition to adulthood during which adolescents complete school, find jobs, and establish families. Only half of the women who give birth before age 18 have finished high school by their mid-20's. Compared with other women, women who give birth as teenagers are less likely to finish either high school or college and are more likely to be unemployed. Those who are employed earn only 50% of the income of women who delay childbearing until at least age 20.[7, 26] These negative social consequences are especially likely to occur among disadvantaged teens in inner cities or rural poverty areas.[12]

Policy and Program Implications

Unintended teenage childbearing remains a problem in the United States. Each year, hundreds of thousands of young girls become mothers by default.[12] The National Academy of Sciences' Panel on Adolescent Pregnancy and Childbearing lists prevention of teen pregnancy as a national priority and asserts that it is less costly to prevent pregnancy than to cope with its consequences.[30] The costs of early childbearing for young families and the larger community represent the failure of a nation to take a preventive approach to teen pregnancy.

The birth rate for school-age mothers reflects a society's commitment to preventing early childbearing. It also reflects the nature and accessibility of family life education; the extent of sexual activity in this age group; the accessibility of contraceptive information, counseling, and services for those who are sexually active; societal emphasis on sexuality and sexual activity; perceived and real options to early parenthood; and the availability and accessibility of safe and legal abortion services.[19, 29]

Status and Trends

National

• Patterns of teenage childbearing in the United States have undergone great change. Both the number of teenagers and the number of children born to them are declining. These facts are reflected in the 1986 teen birth rate of 50.6 per 1,000 for 15- to 19-year-olds—the lowest birth rate for this age group in 50 years[33] (Table 4). Nonetheless, the United States still leads nearly all other developed nations in rates of teenage pregnancy, abortion, and childbearing. In a study of 37 developed countries, the Alan Guttmacher Institute found that the countries with the lowest rates of teenage pregnancy, abortion, and childbearing have the most liberal attitudes toward sex, easily accessible contraceptive services, and effective formal and informal sex education programs.[20]

• According to the National Longitudinal Survey of Work Experience of Youth, only 48% of young American women who first engage in sexual intercourse by age 15 have already had formal sex education; only 26% of their male counterparts have had a sex education course prior to first intercourse.[1, 23]

Table 4. Teen birth rates (births per 1,000 females) by age, race, and marital status: 1980–86.

Population	Age Group		
and Year	10–14	15–17	15–19
All teens			
All races			
1980	1.1	32.5	53.0
1981	1.1	32.1	52.7
1982	1.1	32.4	52.9
1983	1.1	32.0	51.7
1984	1.2	31.1	50.9
1985	1.2	31.1	51.3
1986	1.3	30.6	50.6
Whites			
1980	0.6	25.2	44.7
1981	0.5	25.1	44.6
1982	0.6	25.2	44.6
1983	0.6	24.8	43.6
1984	0.6	23.9	42.5
1985	0.6	24.0	42.8
1986	0.6	23.4	41.8
Blacks			
1980	4.3	73.6	100.0
1981	4.1	70.6	97.1
1982	4.1	71.2	97.0
1983	4.1	70.1	95.5
1984	4.3	69.7	95.7
1985	4.5	69.8	97.4
1986	4.6	70.0	98.1
Unmarried teens			
All Races			
1980		20.6	27.6
1981		20.9	28.2
1982		21.5	28.9
1983		22.1	29.7
1984		21.9	30.2
1985		22.5	31.6
1986		22.9	32.6
Whites			
1980		11.8	16.2
1981		12.4	17.1
1982		12.9	17.7
1983		13.5	18.5
1984		13.5	19.0
1985		14.2	20.5
1986		14.6	21.5
Blacks			
1980		70.6	90.3
1981		69.6	89.2
1982		66.9	86.8
1983		67.6	87.0
1984		66.8	87.1
1985		67.0	88.8
1986		67.4	89.9

Source: National Center for Health Statistics, 1988b.

- According to the National Survey of Family Growth, 46% of all teenage women in the United States have had premarital intercourse, and nearly one-third of those who are sexually active but unmarried have had at least one premarital pregnancy.[11, 30]

- Almost 1 million teens in the United States become pregnant each year; 40% of these pregnancies are aborted and 13% end in miscarriage.[44] In 1986, there were approximately 472,000 births to teens; 6 out of 10 of these births were to unmarried mothers, nearly half of whom (45.8%) had not yet reached their 18th birthday[33] (Table 5).

- The 1986 teen birth rate was 1.3 for adolescents 10 to 14 years old, an 18% increase over the 1980 rate. The 1986 rate was 30.6 per 1,000 for teens 15 to 17 years old[33] (Table 4).

- In 1986, young black women were 7.6 times as likely as young white women to give birth before the age of 15. The birth rate for blacks ages 10 to 14 was 4.6 births per 1,000 young women, compared with a rate of 0.6 for whites in the same age group. Among 15- to 17-year-olds, black teens bear children at a rate nearly three times that of their white counterparts—70.0 versus 23.4 in 1986. Of special concern is that the birth rates for black teens 10 to 14 years old and 15 to 19 years old have increased each year for the past three consecutive years[33] (Table 4).

Table 5. Number of births to teens by age, race, and marital status: 1986

Race and Marital Status	Age Group			
	<20	<15	15–17	18–19
All races	472,081	10,176	168,572	293,333
Married	181,946	761	45,081	136,104
Unmarried	290,135	9,415	123,491	157,229
% Unmarried	61.5%	92.5%	73.2%	53.6%
Whites	315,335	4,007	104,920	206,408
Married	162,210	661	40,855	120,694
Unmarried	153,125	3,346	64,065	85,714
% Unmarried	48.5%	83.5%	61.1%	41.5%
Blacks	141,606	5,877	58,449	77,280
Married	13,594	60	2,735	10,799
Unmarried	128.012	5,817	55,714	66,481
% Unmarried	90.4%	98.9%	95.3%	86%

Source: National Center for Health Statistics, 1988b.

- Overall, teen birth rates declined 26% between 1970 and 1986, from 68.3 per 1,000 teens to 50.6. Between 1980 and 1986, teen birth rates declined 4.5% among 15- to 19-year-olds and 5.8% among 15- to 17-year-olds. In contrast to the general decline in teen birth rates, birth rates among unmarried teens have increased rapidly. Between 1980 and 1986, the birth rate for unmarried teens rose 11% among 15- to 17-year-olds and 18% among 15- to 19-year-olds[33] (Table 4).

- The birth rate for unmarried white teens has tripled since 1970, while the rate among black teens decreased 7.2%.[27] Still, in 1986, the birth rate for unmarried black 15- to 19-year-olds was 4.2 times higher than that for whites.[33] Racial differences are even more pronounced at younger ages. Among unmarried 15- to 17-year-olds, the rate for black teens is 4.6 times the rate for white teens[33] (Table 4).

- Racial disparities in the likelihood of giving birth as a single parent are not primarily attributable to racial differences in rates of premarital sexual activity. Black teens are only slightly more likely than white teens to be sexually active before marriage, but once sexually active, black teens are more likely to become premaritally pregnant, slightly less likely to terminate a premarital pregnancy, and 50% less likely to marry to legitimize a birth.[9, 10, 15, 16, 18, 40]

- In 1986, 12.5% of all births in the United States were to girls in their teens; more than one-third of these births (178,748) were to mothers age 17 or younger (Table 5). That same year, one out of six babies born to Hispanic women were born to teen mothers and nearly 20% of births to American Indian women were to teens.[33]

- Among teens ages 15 to 17, the proportion of births to unmarried mothers increased from 43% in 1970 to 73.2% in 1986.[33, 38] In 1986, in this same age group, 6 out of 10 births to whites and 9 out of 10 births to blacks were to unmarried mothers[33] (Table 5).

- The percentage of teen births to single mothers is growing among Hispanics, as it is among white and black teens. In 1985, 58.5% of births to Hispanic teens were to unmarried mothers. Additionally, 9.3% of babies born to young Hispanic mothers are of low birth weight.[14,33]

- Twenty-five percent of the infants born to mothers under age 15 are premature—a rate three times that of older mothers.[35] In 1986, 15% of all births to mothers younger than 20 years were preterm. Babies born to teenage mothers in 1986 accounted for 17.2% of all LBW infants in the nation. Additionally, 13.8% of births to girls under age 15 and 9.3%

of births to young women ages 15 to 19 were low birth weight, but the rate was 6.0% for women ages 25 to 29.[33]

• The high rates of infant mortality and low birth weight among babies born to teens can be attributed in part to the failure to receive early and continuous high-quality prenatal care.[5] Differences in maternal health and well-being by age may also be due to inadequate prenatal care among adolescents, particularly in the early teen years.[25] In the United States, two out of three pregnant teens under age 15 and almost one-half of teens ages 15 to 17 do not receive prenatal care in the first three months of pregnancy. Additionally, 12.7% of all pregnant teens—one in eight white teens, one in seven Hispanic teens, and one in six black teens—receive late prenatal care or no care at all.[33, 34]

• By age 18, 7% of white teens, 14% of Hispanic teens, and 26% of black teens have given birth. Among young mothers who have their first child before their 18th birthday, 4 out of 10 will have another child within three years.[9]

• In 1986, more than one-third of subsequent births to teenage mothers occurred within 18 months of a previous birth.[33]

• Racial differences in the likelihood of having a repeat birth while still a teen vary by age. In 1986, 6 out of 10 repeat births to teens were to white teens. At ages 15 to 17, black and white teens were equally likely to experience a repeat birth. Among those younger than 15, black teens were twice as likely as white teens to have a repeat birth—66% versus 31%.[28, 33]

State and Local*

• Numbers and rates of teen pregnancies and births vary by state. The states with the highest *numbers* of teen pregnancies and births are not necessarily the states with the highest *rates* of teen pregnancies and births. For instance, the number of babies born to teens in New York in 1985 was six times the number born to teens in New Mexico (25,492 versus 4,232), yet the 1985 teen birth *rate* in New Mexico, 72.4 per 1,000, was almost twice that of New York. Similarly, in 1981 (the most recent year for which state-level pregnancy data are available), the number of teen pregnancies in New York was nearly 10 times the number in New Mexico (80,060 versus 8,340), but the teen pregnancy rate in New Mexico was higher than the rate in New York—131 versus 106 per 1,000 teens.[9, 38]

*The District of Columbia is excluded from the state analyses in this section.

• In 1985, as a percentage of all births, births to teenage women ranged from a low of 7.5% in Minnesota to a high of 20.8% in Mississippi. These two states also ranked highest and lowest among all states in teen birth rates, with Mississippi's high of 78.4 and Minnesota's low of 31.0 per 1,000.[9]

• A 1986 state-by-state analysis of teen pregnancy, birth, and abortion rates reveals that states with high rates of teenage dropouts have high rates of teenage pregnancy and birth and that, in general, high levels of state AFDC payment are not an incentive for early childbearing.[38]

• In 1985, 76 of the 108 largest U.S. cities had percentages of births to teens above the national average. Newark, NJ, had the highest percentage of births to teens (26.3%), and Madison, WI, had the lowest (5.1%).[9]

Risk Factors

Teenage girls without access to effective sex education and appropriate family-planning services run an increased risk of unintended pregnancy. The younger the sexually active teen, the less likely she is to use contraception and the more likely she is to become pregnant. Girls who initiate intercourse prior to age 15 are twice as likely to become pregnant within the first six months as are teens who delay intercourse until ages 18 to 19.[45]

Many of the risks of school-age childbearing are interwoven with its causes and consequences. Low self-esteem and the perception of poor prospects for the future contribute to the risk of early childbearing. Teenagers most at risk of early parenthood are disproportionately those least able to support children: teens from low-income or minority families, those with poor basic skills, those who are failing in school, and those with poor employment potential. Girls with poor basic skills are five times more likely to become mothers before age 16 than those with average basic skills.[8] Whether black, white, or Hispanic, poor young women are three to four times more likely to be unwed mothers than their advantaged counterparts.[14] Additionally, poor teens who already have a child are at increased risk of early repeat pregnancy.[36]

U.S. Objectives for Childbearing Among Young Women

In 1980, the U.S. Department of Health and Human Services set the following objectives for reducing childbearing among young women:

• By 1990, there should be virtually no unintended births to girls 14 years old or younger.

- By 1990, the fertility rate for 15-year-old girls should be reduced to 10 per 1,000.
- By 1990, the fertility rate for 16-year-old girls should be reduced to 25 per 1,000.
- By 1990, the fertility rate for 17-year-old girls should be reduced to 45 per 1,000.[37]

Fulfilling the objective for girls age 14 and younger would reduce births in this age group to near zero. However, in 1986, the number of births to girls under age 15 was higher than it was in 1980[31, 33] (Table 6).

It is not yet certain whether the objectives for 15, 16, and 17-year-olds will be reached by 1990; birth rates for these ages were 13.4, 30.1, and 49.8, respectively, in 1984.[31]

Data Sources

State and Local

The state's vital statistics registrar is responsible for collecting data from birth certificates before the data are sent to NCHS and can provide state and local data on births to teenagers. Most states publish birth data annually. Some states can provide data by census tract, which is one means of estimating the socioeconomic status of the family. In large cities, the office of vital statistics in the city or county health department may publish its own data.

Table 6. Number of births to women younger than age 15: 1978–86 and U.S. 1990 Objective.

Year	No. Births
1978	10,772
1979	10,669
1980	10,169
1981	9,632
1982	9,773
1983	9,752
1984	9,965
1985	10,220
1986	10,176
1990 Objective	10,176

Source: National Center for Health Statistics 1986, 1988b.

National

Vital Statistics of the Unites States, Vol. I, Natality, published annually by the NCHS, is a good source of national data on births to young teenagers. Based on birth certificate data from the VSRS, this volume provides information on births to young women under age 15 and ages 15, 16, and 17, tabulated by race of infant, birth weight, birth order, mother's marital status, interval since last birth, and number of prenatal visits. Volume III of the same publication contains data on marriages classified by characteristics of the bride and groom, including age and race. It takes approximately three to four years before the birth and marriage data for a calendar year are published.

A more timely, but less complete source of final national data (one-to two-year lag) is the NCHS *Advance Report of Final Natality Statistics,* part of the Monthly Vital Statistics Report series. The *Advance Report* provides data on the number of live births and birth rates by age group, live birth order, and race of child; trend data on fertility rates and birth rates by age of mother and race of child; data on the number and percentage of LBW infants by birth weight, age of mother, and race of child; and data on prenatal care by age of mother and race of child. The *Advance Report of Final Marriage Statistics* provides final data on marriages of teens.

Provisional data on births and marriages are published (two- to three-month lag) in *Births, Marriages, Divorces and Deaths.* This publication is also a part of the Monthly Vital Statistics Report series.

In the Monthly Vital Statistics Report series, NCHS also reports abortion ratios by age, race, marital status, and educational attainment for selected states. These data appear in *Induced Terminations of Pregnancy: Reporting States.* The most recent publication contains 1982–83 data for 13 states.

The National Natality Follow-Back Surveys (NNS) are a source of data on births to young women tabulated by characteristics other than those reported on birth certificates. Conducted by NCHS in 1963–69, 1972, and 1980, these surveys include birth information by characteristics such as mother's occupation and work history during pregnancy, father's occupation, source of medical care for mother and infant, family income, mother's smoking and drinking habits, and whether the baby is breast- or bottle-fed. NCHS publishes data from the NNS periodically in the Vital and Health Statistics series.

Reliable and detailed information on teenage childbearing is available every 10 years from the Decennial Census. The special value of the Decennial Census data is that they provide information on fertility characteristics of teenagers, such as number of births, number of premarital births, and number of premarital conceptions, and can be used to make accurate estimates for small geographic divisions and for various population groups. The obvious disadvantage of Census data is that they are collected only every 10 years. The Bureau of the Census estimates the size of the population for states and localities for non-Census years (rounded to the nearest thousand), but it provides only limited population breakdowns. Estimates are available by age, race, or sex, but not by all three variables at once. Thus, it is possible to obtain estimates of the number of women, the number of teenagers, or the number of Hispanics in the United States, but not the number of Hispanic teenage women or even the number of teenage women.

Information on specific characteristics of women ages 15, 16, and 17 is also available through the National Survey of Family Growth (NSFG), Cycle III, conducted by NCHS in 1982. Cycle III provides data on background characteristics of the mother, such as fertility, family planning, prenatal care, and pregnancy outcome; the short-term health status of the child; and level of sex education and characteristics of the sexually active population as a whole. Data are reported by age (in single years and in five-year age groups), race, and marital status. The survey results are available on public-use data tapes through the National Technical Information Service. In addition, the results of the survey are being published in 12 installments in series 23 of *Vital and Health Statistics*. A new NSFG cycle began in 1988.

National estimates of sexual activity and contraception are available from the National Surveys of Young Women and Men (1971, 1976, and 1979). These three surveys, conducted by John Kanter and Melvin Zelnick at Johns Hopkins University, included 15- to 19-year-old women; the 1979 survey also included 17- to 21-year-old men.

Finally, the CDC and the Alan Guttmacher Institute (AGI) report estimates of rates of teenage pregnancy. The most recent CDC summary reports data for 1970, 1974, and 1980 and is available as a supplement to the *Morbidity and Mortality Weekly Report*. The most recent published data from AGI are for 1981; unpublished tabulations for more recent years are available directly from AGI.

Data Needs

National

There is a three-year lag between the end of a calendar year and publication of final national data for that year. This relatively long lag precludes use of timely data for evaluating, planning, and implementing public policies and programs.

There is a great need in the current national data system to develop a mechanism to link birth and death records. This linkage would allow an analysis of the relationship between births to young women under age 18 and infant mortality. Efforts are currently under way to address this relationship through an NCHS pilot program to develop an ongoing national file on linked birth and death certificates, starting with the 1982 and 1983 birth cohorts, and through a CDC program to compile data from linked birth and death certificates from individual states, beginning with the 1980 birth cohort.

Another limitation of national data on births to teenagers is the paucity of information on the well-being of the children of young mothers and an immediate and long-term impact of early childbearing on the parents. A regular series of data on the health and socioeconomic conditions of young mothers as they age and of their children would be useful for longitudinal analysis.

National data collected by ethnicity are not complete. National data on births to teenage women of Hispanic origin were first available for the 1978 cohort, based on reporting from 17 states. The 1985 data on Hispanics are based on reporting from 23 states and the District of Columbia. NCHS computes the birth rate for Hispanic teenagers by using the number of live births in the 23 reporting states.[34] However, birth rates are not computed for intercensal years, as population data are unreliable. NCHS first published data on births to young women of Asian origin (Chinese, Filipino, Japanese, Hawaiian, etc.) in 1984.[42]

References

1. Adams-Taylor S, Morich M, Pittman K, Adams G. What about the boys?: teenage pregnancy prevention strategies. Adolescent Pregnancy Prevention Clearinghouse Report (Jul). Washington, DC: Children's Defense Fund, 1988.

2. Alan Guttmacher Institute. Teenage pregnancy: the problem that hasn't gone away. New York: Alan Guttmacher Institute, 1981.

3. Alan Guttmacher Institute. Teens get poor prenatal care: their babies are at greater risk of death. Family Planning Perspectives 1982;14(May–Jun):146–7.

4. Alan Guttmacher Institute. Children born to teens more likely to be injured or hospitalized by age 5. Family Planning Perspectives 1983;16(Sep–Oct):238.

5. Baldwin W, Cain V. The children of teenage parents. In: Furstenberg F, Lincoln R, Menken J, eds. Teenage sexuality, pregnancy, and childbearing. Philadelphia: University of Pennsylvania Press, 1981;265–79.

6. Brooks-Gunn J, Furstenberg F. Children of adolescent mothers: physical, academic and psychological outcomes. Developmental Review 1986;6:224–51.

7. Children's Defense Fund. When children have children: teens with infants face an uphill battle. CDF Reports 1984;6(Jun).

8. Children's Defense Fund. Preventing adolescent pregnancy: what schools can do. Adolescent Pregnancy Prevention Chearinghouse Report (Sep). Washington, DC: Children's Defense Fund, 1986.

9. Children's Defense Fund. Teenage pregnancy: an advocate's guide to the numbers. Adolescent Pregnancy Prevention Clearinghouse Report Series (Jan–Mar). Washington, DC: Children's Defense Fund, 1988.

10. Cutright P, Smith HL. Intermediate determinants of racial differences in 1980 U.S. nonmarital fertility rates. Family Planning Perspectives 1988;20(May–Jun):119–23.

11. Dawson DA. The effects of sex education on adolescent behavior. Family Planning Perspectives 1986;18(Jul–Aug):162–70.

12. Dryfoos J. A time for new thinking about teenage pregnancy. American Journal of Public Health 1985;75(1):13–4.

13. Edelman MW, Pittman KJ. Adolescent pregnancy: black and white. Journal Community Health 1986;2(Spring):63–9.

14. Fennelly K. El embarazo precoz: Childbearing amont Hispanic teenagers in the United States. New York: Columbia University Press, 1988.

15. Flick LH. Paths to adolescent parenthood: implications for prevention. Public Health Reports 1986;101(Mar–Apr):132–47.

16. Furstenberg F. Race differences in teenage sexuality, pregnancy, and adolescent childbearing. The Milbank Quarterly 1987;65(Supplement 2):381–403.

17. Furstenberg F, Brooks-Gunn J, Morgan SP. Adolescent mothers in later life. New York: Cambridge University Press, 1987.

18. Hofferth SL, Kahn JR, Baldwin W. Premarital sexual activity among US teenage women over the past three decades. Family Planning Perspectives 1987;19(Mar–Apr):46–53.

19. Hogan D, Alstone N, Kitagawa E. Social and environmental factors influencing contraceptive use among black adolescents. Family Planning Perspectives 1985;17(Jul–Aug):165–9.

20. Jones E, Forrest J, Goldman N, Henshaw S, Lincoln B, Rosoff J, Westoff C, Wulf D. Teenage pregnancy in developed countries: determinants and policy implications. Family Planning Perspectives 1985;17(Mar–Apr):53–63.

21. Levanthal J. Risk factors for child abuse: methodologic standards in case-control studies. Pediatrics 1981;68(5):684–90.

22. Makinson C. The health consequences of teenage fertility. Family Planning Perspectives 1985;17(May–Jun):132–9.

23. Marsiglio W, Mott FL. The impact of sex education on sexual activity, contraceptive use and premarital pregnancy among American teenagers. Family Planning Perspectives 1986;18(Jul–Aug):151–61.

24. McAnarney E. Young maternal age and adverse neonatal outcome. AJDC 1987;141(Oct):1053–8.

25. McAnarney E, Thiede H. Adolescent pregnancy and childbearing: what we learned during the 1970s and what remains to be learned. In: McAnarney ER, ed. Premature adolescent pregnancy and parenthood. New York: Grune and Stratton, 1983.

26. Menken J. The health and social consequences of teenage childbearing. In: Furstenberg F, Lincoln R, Menken J, eds. Teenage sexuality, pregnancy, and childbearing. Philadelphia: University of Pennsylvania Press, 1981:167–83.

27. Moore K, Simms M, Betsey C. Choice and circumstance: racial differences in adolescent sexuality and fertility. New Brunswick, NJ: Transaction Books, 1986.

28. Mott FL. The pace of repeated childbearing among young American mothers. Family Planning Perspectives 1986;18(Jan–Feb):5–11.

29. Nathanson C, Becker M. The influences of client-provider relationships on teenage women's subsequent use of contraception. American Journal of Public Health 1985;75(Jan):33–8.

30. National Academy of Sciences. Risking the future: adolescent sexuality, pregnancy, and childbearing. Two Volumes. Washington, DC: National Academy Press, 1987.

31. National Center for Health Statistics. Health, United States and prevention profile, 1986. DHHS Pub. No. (PHS)87–1232. Washington, DC: NCHS, 1986.

32. National Center for Health Statistics. Advance report of final natality statistics, 1985. Monthly Vital Statistics Report 36(Jul). DHHS Pub. No. (PHS)87–1120. Washington, DC: NCHS, 1986.

33. National Center for Health Statistics. Advance report of final natality statistics, 1986. Monthly Vital Statistics Report 37(Jul). DHHS Pub. No. (PHS)88–1120. Washington, DC: NCHS, 1988.

34. National Center for Health Statistics. Births of Hispanic parentage. Monthly Vital Statistics Report 36(Feb). DHHS Pub. No. (PHS)88–1120. Washington, DC: NCHS, 1988.

35. Petit M, Overcash D. America's children: powerless and in need of powerful friends. Augusta, ME: Maine Department of Public Health, 1983.

36. Polit D, Kahn J. Early subsequent pregnancy among economically disadvantaged teenage mothers. American Journal of Public Health 1986;76(Feb):167–71.

37. Public Health Service. Promoting health/preventing disease: objectives for the nation. DHHS Pub. No. (OM)81–0007. Washington, DC: PHS, 1980.

38. Singh S. Adolescent pregnancy in the United States: an interstate analysis. Family Planning Perspectives 1986; 18(Sep–Oct):210–20.

39. Southern Regional Project on Infant Mortality. Adolescent pregnancy in the South. Washington, DC: Southern Governors' Association, 1988.

40. Stephan S. Teenage pregnancy and childbearing: incidence data. Congressional Research Service Report No. (EPW)87–11. Washington, DC: Library of Congress, 1987.

41. Strobino D. The health and medical consequences of adolescent sexuality and pregnancy: a review of the literature. In: Hayes C, ed. Risking the future: adolescent sexuality, pregnancy, and childbearing: vol II, Working papers and statistical appendixes. Washington, DC: National Adademy Press, 1987.

42. Taffel S. Characteristics of Asian births: United States, 1980. Monthly Vital Statistics Report 32(10). DHHS Pub. No. (PHS)84–1120. Washington, DC: National Center for Health Statistics, 1984.

43. Ventura S, Hendershot G. Infant health consequences of childbearing by teenagers and older mothers. Public Health Reports, 1984;99(2):138–46.

44. Ventura S, Taffel S, Mosher W. Estimates of pregnancies and pregnancy rates for the United States, 1976–1985. American Journal of Public Health 1988;78(May):506–11.

45. Zabin L, Kantner J, Zelnick M. The risk of adolescent pregnancy in the first months of intercourse. In: Furstenberg F, Lincoln R, Menken J, eds. Teenage sexuality, pregnancy, and childbearing. Philadelphia: University of Pennsylvania Press, 1981:136–48.

Suicides

Definition

Suicide is the intentional taking of one's own life.

Indicator

* The number of suicides among youths ages 15 to 24 years within a defined population.

Significance

Health Implications

Suicide among the young is a major U.S. public health riddle and a leading cause of unnecessary, preventable, and stigmatizing death.[11] For people who attempt suicide and fail, the result can be permanent mental or physical disability as well as continuing emotional stress. The most frequent methods of suicide—poisoning by solids, liquids, or gases; hanging and strangulation; drowning; firearms and explosives; cutting and piercing wounds; and jumping—all carry grave dangers for survivors, such as brain damage due to lack of oxygen, broken bones, spinal cord injury, nerve damage, and malfunctioning of the liver, kidneys, and other internal organs.[9, 12]

Policy and Program Implications

Each suicide by a child or youth is an event that should not have occurred. Attempts to address the issue of suicide among youths must involve a strong commitment to improve mental health.

Statistics tell the story of the growing proportion of young people who are not able to find their way toward mature social adjustment. A high incidence of suicides by youths within a defined population reflects inadequacies in social support systems, health services, and socioeconomic opportunities that help promote survival and emotional well-being.

The extent to which suicide is influenced by biologic factors is unknown. Present knowledge suggests that a high incidence of suicide among children and youths implies the need for (1) intervention programs aimed at reducing socioeconomic and emotional stresses, (2) improved recognition and treatment of depression, (3) counseling and support programs for adolescents at risk for suicide, (4) interventions aimed at reducing access to suicide methods, and (5) improved access to poison control information by telephone and in hospital emergency rooms.

Status and Trends

• Suicide is the second leading cause of death in the United States among 15- to 24-year-olds. In 1985, more than 5,000 adolescents and young adults took their own lives, resulting in a suicide rate of 12.9 per 100,000 young people.[14]

• Suicide among today's youth is a growing problem. From 1970 to 1985, the suicide rate among 15- to 24-year-olds increased 46% (from 8.8 to 12.9 per 100,000). This increase was due primarily to a 56% increase in the suicide rate among males. The rate for females in this age group increased only 2%[4, 15] (Figure 6).

• Suicide rates among 20- to 24-year olds, although still considerably higher than the rates among teens, decreased for the sexes, races, and race/sex combinations from 1980 to 1985. This same period witnessed alarmingly persistent increases in the rate of suicide among younger age groups. Since 1980, the suicide rate among 15- to 19-year-olds increased

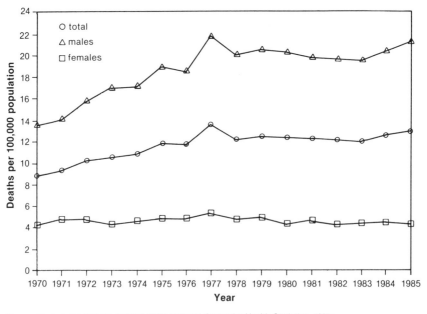

Source: Centers for Disease Control, 1987; National Center for Health Statistics, 1987c.

Figure 6. Suicide rates among youths ages 15 to 24 by gender, 1970–85.

17.6% (8.5 in 1980, 10.0 in 1985), while the rate among 10- to 14-year-olds doubled[17] (Table 7).

• Among 15- to 24-year-olds, the suicide rate for whites is nearly twice that for blacks (13.8 per 100,000 vs. 7.6 per 100,000). A closer look, however, reveals more variation in the rate for blacks than for whites. From 1984 to 1985, the suicide rate for white males increased 3% (22.0 to 22.7), while the rate for white females remained stable (4.7). During the same period, the suicide rate for black males increased 18.7% (11.2 to 13.3), and the rate for black females decreased 16.6% (2.4 to 2.0)[15] (Table 8).

• From 1960 to 1985, among 15- to 24-year-olds, the suicide rate tripled for black males and almost doubled for black females. Trends among white males and females were similar. In 1985, the suicide rate among black males in this age group was more than six times the rate for black females, a ratio that has doubled since 1960[15] (Table 8).

Table 7. Suicide rates (number per 100,000 population) by age, sex, and race: 1980 and 1985.

Population	Year	Age Group					
		10–14		15–19		20–24	
		Rate	Change (%)	Rate	Change (%)	Rate	Change (%)
Total	1980	0.8		8.5		16.1	
	1985	1.6	100.0	10.0	17.6	15.6	− 3.1
Males	1980	1.2		13.8		26.8	
	1985	2.3	91.6	16.0	15.9	26.2	− 2.2
Whites	1980	1.4		15.0		27.8	
	1985	2.5	78.5	17.3	15.3	27.4	− 1.4
Blacks	1980	0.5		5.6		20.0	
	1985	1.3	16.0	8.2	46.4	18.5	− 7.5
Females	1980	0.3		3.0		5.5	
	1985	0.9	200.0	3.7	23.3	4.9	− 10.9
Whites	1980	0.3		3.3		5.9	
	1985	0.9	200.0	4.1	24.2	5.2	− 11.9
Blacks	1980	0.1		1.6		3.1	
	1985	0.4	300.0	1.5	6.3	2.4	− 22.5

Source: National Center for Health Statistics, 1987b.

Table 8. Suicide rates (number per 100,000 population) among 15- to 24-year-olds by race and sex: 1960–85.

Year	White Males	White Females	Black Males	Black Females
1985	22.7	4.7	13.3	2.0
1984	22.0	4.7	11.2	2.4
1983	20.6	4.6	11.5	2.7
1982	21.2	4.5	11.0	2.2
1981	21.1	4.9	11.1	2.4
1980	21.4	4.6	12.3	2.3
1975	19.3	4.9	12.7	3.2
1970	13.9	4.2	10.5	3.8
1965	9.5	2.9	8.1	2.5
1960	8.6	2.3	4.1	1.3

Source: National Center for Health Statistics, 1987c.

• For all race and sex categories the highest suicide rate for 15- to 24-year-olds is among white males (22.7 per 100,000). Young white males committed suicide at a rate 4.8 times the rate for white females, 1.7 times the rate for black males, and 11.4 times the rate for black females[15] (Table 8).

• Suicide rates among 15- to 24-year-old Hispanics have tripled in the past three decades. However, a recent five-year study of suicide rates among Hispanics in five Southwestern states revealed that Hispanic males and females are at less risk for suicide than whites.[22]

• Suicide rates among 15- to 24-year-old American Indian and Alaskan Native Reservation populations, although exceptionally high, have been decreasing. Rates for this age group were 32.6 per 100,000 in 1970, 30.3 in 1980, and 27.9 in 1982.[20]

• Teenage and young adult males committed suicide at a rate almost five times that of females in 1985 (21.4 vs. 4.4).[15]

• Youths make an estimated half a million serious suicide attempts each year. Females are more likely than males to attempt suicide, whereas males are more likely than females to complete suicide.[3, 8, 18]

• Among youths who attempt suicide and fail, an estimated 6% to 16% will attempt again within one year. Repeat episodes of attempted suicide are more common among adolescent females.[5, 23]

• The rate of use of firearms to commit suicide has increased dramatically since 1970 among 15- to 24-year-old males.[2, 20] In 1985, 62% of young men in this age group used firearms to kill themselves. Of the various methods of suicide, males were most likely to use firearms and hanging. Females were 5.4 times more likely to use drugs and 1.6 times more likely to use gas to commit suicide than were males[16] (Table 9).

Risk Factors

The lack of readily available study and control subjects and difficulties associated with obtaining unbiased, comparable information on all subjects hinder the identification of risk factors for suicide. Nonetheless, several predisposing factors can be identified. Children, youths, and young adults at increased risk of committing suicide include those with a history of major psychiatric disorder, drug or alcohol abuse, recent behavioral changes such as depression or truancy, previous suicide attempts, or suicide by a family member.[1, 24]

Table 9. Number and distribution of suicides among 15- to 24-year-olds by method: 1985.

Method	Number of Suicides			Percentage of total for all causes		
	Total	Males	Females	Total	Males	Females
Handguns and all other firearms	3081	2650	431	60.2	62.1	50.5
Hanging, strangulation, and suffocation	970	864	106	18.9	20.2	12.4
Gases and vapors	444	338	106	8.7	7.9	12.4
Drugs, medicaments, and biologicals	293	141	152	5.7	3.3	17.8
Other solids and liquids	36	30	6	0.7	0.7	0.7
All other causes	297	244	53	5.8	5.7	6.2
All causes	5121	4267	854	100	100	100

Source: National Center for Health Statistics, 1987d.
Calculations by Child Health Outcomes Project.

Also associated with increased risk of suicide among children and youths are divorce or separation of parents, unwanted pregnancy among adolescents, and other stressful situations, such as problems with romance, loss of a parent or other significant relative, sense of failure, or recent humiliation or punishment,[7, 12, 21, 24] For those who have expressed intent to commit suicide, the continued availability of firearms or other means of suicide poses an increased risk as well.[2, 6]

U.S. Objective for Reducing the Suicide Rate among Young People

The U.S. Department of Health and Human Services established the following objective for reducing suicides among youths:
- By 1990, the rate of suicide among people ages 15 to 24 should be below 11 per 100,000.[19]

In 1978, the suicide rate for this age group was 12.1 per 100,000, but the rate has increased 6.6% from this baseline. In fact, with the exception of 1983, the rate of suicide for this age group has been the same as or higher than the rate for the year the objective was established[13] (Silverman et al. 1988) (Figure 7).

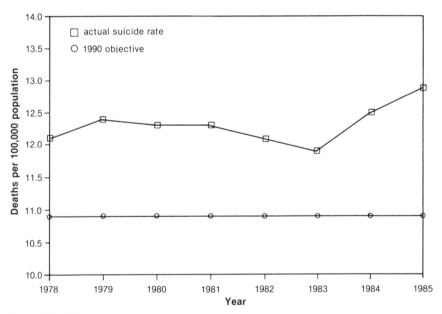

Source: National Center for Health Statistics, 1986, 1987a.

Figure 7. Suicide rates among youths ages 15 to 24, 1978–85 and U.S. 1990 Objective.

A number of factors will influence this nation's ability to halt spiraling suicide rates among this age group, including the forthcoming recommendations of the U.S. Department of Health and Human Services Secretary's Task Force on Youth Suicide. Present trends indicate that the suicide rate among 15- to 24-year-olds will continue to increase markedly into the next century unless a significant nationwide intervention program is developed and policy directions shifted.[10]

Data Sources

State and Local

The registrar of vital statistics at the state, city, or county department of health can provide the most timely state and local data on suicides. This information is extracted from death certificates at the state level before being sent to the National Center for Health Statistics (NCHS) for tabulation.

National

NCHS publishes the most complete national data on suicide in *Vital Statistics of the United States, Vol. II, Mortality*. Based on data the VSRS extracts from death certificates, this volume provides information on incidence of suicide by age group (5–9, 10–14, 15–19 years), race (black, white, and all other), sex, and method used (poisoning by drugs or medicaments; poisoning by other solid or liquid substances; poisoning by gases or vapors; hanging, strangulation, or suffocation; firearms or explosives; and all other means). There is about a two- to three-year lag between the end of a calendar year and publication of data for that year.

A more timely, but less comprehensive source of data is the *Advance Report of Final Mortality Statistics*, part of the Monthly Vital Statistics Report series. This report provides data on the number of suicides and suicide rates by 10-year age groups. Data are published approximately two years after the end of the calendar year.

Data Needs

National

Several methodological shortcomings become apparent when utilizing our current national data systems to analyze suicide rates among children, adolescents, and young adults. The social stigma and guilt surrounding suicide in childhood and adolescence may contribute to the "covering up" of suicides by parents, family physicians, and others, resulting in underreporting of suicides on death certificates. Additional underreporting may result when, because of the absence of a note or other evidence, suicides are labeled accidents.

On the national level, changes in classification for suicide also contribute to methodological problems in analysis. Revisions over time in the International Classification of Diseases can result in discontinuities, as the suicide mortality rate may differ from one revision to the next solely because of reclassification of deaths. The extent of comparability between revisions should be considered in order to differentiate real changes in mortality rates from artifact.

Timely suicide data cannot be used for planning, implementing, and evaluating prevention programs and public policies because of the lag between the end of a calendar year and publication of final national data for that year.

National data by race and ethnicity are limited. Neither rates nor numbers of suicides among Hispanic-origin children and adolescents are available from NCHS (Hispanic-origin question added to death certificate in 1978). Suicide rates for American Indian, Chinese, and Japanese populations are currently not published; however, unpublished data on the number of suicides for each group can be obtained from NCHS.

References

1. Allen BP. Youth suicide. Adolescence 1987;22(Summer):271–90.

2. Boyd J, Moscicki E. Firearms and youth suicide. Am J Public Health 1986;76(Oct): 1240–2.

3. Centers for Disease Control. Suicide—United States. 1970–1980. MMWR 1985;34(21 Jun):353–7.

4. Centers for Disease Control. Youth suicide—United States, 1970–1980. MMWR 1987;36(Jun):87–9.

5. Deykin E, Perlow R, McNamara J. Non-fatal suicidal and life-threatening behavior among 13–17 year old adolescents seeking emergency care. Am J Public Health 1985;75:90–2.

6. Eisenberg L. Adolescent suicide: on taking arms against a sea of troubles. Pediatrics 1980;66(Aug):315–20.

7. Fine P, McIntire M, Fain P. Early indications of self-destruction in childhood and adolescence. Pediatrics 1986;77(Apr):557–68.

8. Hawton K, Catalan J. Attempted suicide. New York: Oxford University Press, 1987.

9. Holinger P. Adolescent suicide: an epidemiological study of recent trends. Am J Psychiatry 1978;135(Jun):754–6.

10. Holinger P, Offer O. Toward the prediction of violent deaths among the young. In: Sudak H, Ford A, Rushforth N, eds. Suicide in the young. Ceton, MA: John Wright, 1984.

11. McGinnis JM. Suicide in America—moving up the public health agenda. Suicide and Life-Threatening Behavior 1987;17(Spring):18–32.

12. McIntire M. The epidemiology and taxonomy of suicide. In: McIntire M, Angle C, eds. Suicide attempts in children and youth. Hagerstown, MD: Harper and Row, 1980.

13. National Center for Health Statistics. Health—United States 1986 and prevention profile. DHHS Pub. No. (PHS)87-1232. Washington, DC: NCHS, 1986.

14. National Center for Health Statistics. Advance report of final mortality statistics, 1985. Monthly Vital Statistics Report 36(Aug), Supplement. DHHS Pub. No. (PHS)87-1120. Washington, DC: NCHS, 1987.

15. National Center for Health Statistics. Deaths and death rates from suicide for ages 15-24 years, by race and sex: United States, 1960-1985. Unpublished data. 1987.

16. National Center for Health Statistics. Table 292. deaths for 282 selected causes by five-year age groups, color and sex, United States, 1979-85. Unpublished data. 1987.

17. National Center for Health Statistics. Table 292-A. death rates for 282 selected causes by five-year age groups, color and sex: United States, 1979-1985. Unpublished data. 1987.

18. Peck M, Farberow N, Litman R. Youth suicide. New York: Springer, 1985.

19. Public Health Service. Promoting health/preventing disease: objectives for the nation. DHHS Pub. No. (OM)81-0007. Washington, DC: PHS, 1980.

20. Silverman TC, Rosenberg M, Smith J, Parron D, Jacobs J. Control of stress and violent behavior: mid-course review of the 1990 Health Objectives. Public Health Reports 1988;103(Jan–Feb):39–48.

21. Smith J, Carter J. Suicide and black adolescents: a medical dilemma. J National Medical Assoc 1986;78(Nov):1061–4.

22. Smith J, Mercy J, Rosenberg M. Suicide and homicide among Hispanics in the Southwest. Public Health Reports 1986,101(May–Jun):265–70.

23. Stephens BJ. Cheap thrills and humble pie: the adolescence of female suicide attempters. Suicide and Life-Threatening Behaviors 1987;17(Summer):107–18.

24. Waldron I, Eyer J. Socioeconomic causes of the recent rise in death rates for 15-24 year olds. Soc Sci Med 1975;9:383–96.

Motor Vehicle Accident Fatalities

Definition

A motor vehicle accident fatality is a death resulting from a motor vehicle accident, whether the victim is a passenger, pedestrian, cyclist, or driver.

Indicator

• The rate of motor vehicle accident fatalities (deaths per 100,000 population) for the following age groups: under 1, 1–4, 5–14, and 15–19.

Significance

Health Implications

According to the National Health Interview Survey, in 1985, motor vehicle accidents injured more than 5 million people in the United States, were a major source of activity restriction and bed-disability, and cost the nation more than $50 billion.[7,15] These accidents are responsible for the largest proportion of intracranial and internal injuries to children and youths. Children who survive potentially fatal motor vehicle accidents may suffer severe, permanent physical or mental damage requiring extensive treatment or extended care.

Policy and Program Implications

As a nation, we have generally made great strides in preventing or reducing childhood deaths from various diseases. However, similar progress has not occurred in reducing the rate of motor vehicle accident fatalities during childhood and adolescence. Although legislative, regulatory, educational, and other initiatives have met with some success, motor vehicle accidents remain a major cause of premature and, largely, preventable death.

The rate of motor vehicle fatalities is a measure of the adequacy or inadequacy of a broad range of public health interventions, including the implementation and enforcement of programs and policies requiring or facilitating use of safety restraints for auto passengers (including infants) and helmets for cyclists; improving the safety design of vehicles and highways; lowering the maximum speed limit; developing alternative bike paths; and raising the legal age for drinking or driving or both, imposing more stringent penalties on drunk drivers, and taking other measures that reduce the incidence of driving under the influence of drugs or alcohol.

Status and Trends

National

• During 1985, nearly 46,000 people died in the United States as a result of motor vehicle accidents; 21% of these people were 19 years of age and under.[10]

• Accidents are the leading cause of death among people ages 1 to 19 years. In 1985, more than 8 out of 10 deaths in this age group were due to accidents, and motor vehicle accidents specifically accounted for 56% of the deaths in this age group[9, 10] (Figure 8).

• Sporadic declines in the rate of motor vehicle deaths among teens have occurred in the past two decades. Nonetheless, in 1985, more than 40% of all deaths among 15- to 19-year olds were the result of motor vehicle accidents, producing a death rate of 33.9 per 100,000. This rate was more than three times the 10.0 rate for suicide, the second leading cause of death for this age group.[9, 10, 11]

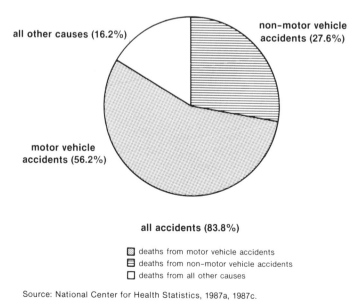

Figure 8. Cause of death for children ages 1 to 19, 1985.

• The death rate for motor vehicle accidents declined approximately 26% between 1980 and 1985 for children younger than age 20. However, the rate increased between 1984 and 1985 for each five-year childhood age group except 15- to 19-year-olds, who experienced a 2% decline[11] (Table 10). The National Highway Traffic Safety Administration (NHTSA) notes that young adults aged 18 to 20 had the most significant decline in the rate of motor vehicle accident fatalities; the rate decreased nearly 8% between 1984 and 1985 in this age group.

• Death rates for various kinds of motor vehicle accidents show distinctive patterns by age: the peak death rates for pedestrians are at ages 6 and 18; for bicyclists, ages 11 to 15; for automobile occupants, ages 18 to 20; and for motorcyclists, ages 18 to 22.[1]

• Males continue to outnumber females as victims of fatal motor vehicle accidents, with the disparity increasing in each childhood age group. In 1985, the rate of motor vehicle accident fatalities for male infants was about the same as that for female infants, but the rate for males was 2.3 times the rate for females among 15- to 19-year-olds[11] (Figure 9).

• During the teenage years, white males have by far the highest rate of death from motor vehicle accidents (51.9 per 100,000 for 15- to 19-year-olds in 1985) compared with black males and both white and black females. Among teens between 15 and 19 years of age, white males die from motor vehicle accidents at 2.4 times the rate of black males, 2.3 times the rate of white females, and 7.0 times the rate of black females.[11]

• Gender differences aside, teenagers are responsible for five times as many crash deaths per license holder as drivers ages 35 to 64.[19]

Table 10. Rates of motor vehicle accident fatalities (number per 100,000 population) by age: 1980-85.

Year	Age Group				
	<1	1-4	5-9	10-14	15-19
1980	7.0	9.2	7.6	8.1	43.0
1981	6.1	7.8	7.4	7.6	39.0
1982	5.8	7.9	6.5	7.0	35.0
1983	5.2	7.5	6.4	6.8	33.2
1984	4.4	6.9	6.2	7.1	34.6
1985	4.8	7.1	6.3	7.3	33.9

Source: National Center for Health Statistics, 1987b.

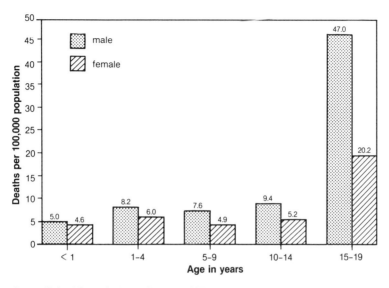

Source: National Center for Health Statistics, 1987b.

Figure 9. Rates of motor vehicle accident fatalities by age and sex, 1985.

• An analysis of rates of motor vehicle accident fatalities by race shows an age-related trend. In 1985, white 15- to 19-year olds died at a rate 4.3 times that of their black peers, and white adolescents died at 2.3 times the rate of black adolescents. Black and white youngsters aged 1 to 4 and 5 to 9 died at nearly equal rates, but black infants died at a rate nearly twice that of white infants[11] (Figure 10).

• Fatality rates for motor vehicle occupants are almost three times higher in low-income areas than in areas with higher per capita income. Poorer roads, older vehicles, and poorer emergency and medical care all contribute to the higher death rates. Additionally, teenage drivers in high-income areas use seat belts at more than three times the rate of teenage drivers in low-income areas.[1, 21]

• Restrained children are 50% to 70% less likely to be injured or killed in an auto accident than unrestrained children.[12] The rate of restraint usage for children younger than age five rose from 6% in 1980 to 40% in 1986. Children who survived an auto accident were more likely to have been restrained than those who died—45% versus 26%.[14]

• The National Health Interview Survey reports only one-third of all children under age seven use seat belts regularly. The survey also reports low usage rates among young mothers, Hispanics, and blacks.[5]

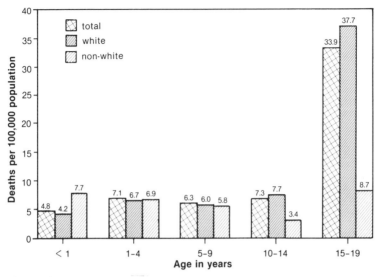

Source: National Center for Health Statistics, 1987b.

Figure 10. Rates of motor vehicle accident fatalities by age and race, 1985.

• Alcohol is a contributing factor in approximately 20% of all crashes resulting in an injury, 50% of all fatal crashes, and 60% of all fatal crashes involving a single vehicle.[6] In 1985, 3860 children under age 20 died in alcohol-related motor vehicle accidents.[13]

• Among 16- to 19-year-old drivers in fatal motor vehicle accidents, the proportion who were intoxicated has decreased in recent years. In 1982, 29% of teenage drivers in fatal crashes were determined to be drunk, compared with 20% in 1985.[13]

State and Local

• As of July 1, 1986, 26 states and the District of Columbia had enacted laws requiring use of seat belts. These laws are generally associated with increases in the use of seat belts and decreases in fatalities.[20] In the six states that implemented usage laws in early 1985—New York, New Jersey, Illinois, Michigan, Texas, and Nebraska—declines in fatalities have saved nearly 525 lives.[20]

• All 50 states and the District of Columbia have implemented laws requiring use of restraints for young children in automobiles. As a result of such laws, Michigan witnessed a 25% decrease in the number of children under age four injured in crashes,[18] and New Mexico experienced a 33% reduction in fatality rates and a 13% reduction in injury rates for children younger than age five.[17]

• As of July 1987, 48 states and the District of Columbia had laws making 21 the legal age for drinking or purchasing alcohol.[15] In a 26-state study of fatal crashes, raising the minimum legal age for purchasing alcohol produced a 13% reduction in nighttime driver fatalities.[4]

• At one time nearly all states had enacted statutes requiring motorcyclists to wear helmets. These laws have been rescinded in many states in response to lobbying on behalf of "personal freedoms."

Risk Factors

Among children and youths, adolescent males are at greatest risk of dying in a motor vehicle accident. Experimentation with alcohol, combined with driving inexperience, increases teenagers' risk of being involved in fatal motor vehicle accidents.[2]

For auto passengers under age 13, infants are at greatest risk. For all age groups, the use of auto safety restraints dramatically decreases the risk of motor vehicle accident fatality, as does use of a helmet for cyclists.

U.S. Objective for Reducing Motor Vehicle Fatalities

In 1980, the U.S. Department of Health and Human Services set the following objective for reducing motor vehicle fatalities among children and youths:

• By 1990, the rate of motor vehicle fatalities for children under age 15 should be reduced to no greater than 5.5 per 100,000 children.[16]

In 1978, the rate of motor vehicle accident fatalities for this age group was 9.0 per 100,000, and the rate declined steadily from 1978 to 1984. However, the 1985 rate of 6.9 per 100,000 represents a 4.5% increase over the 1984 fatality rate of 6.6 per 100,000 (Figure 4). Motor vehicle injuries accounted for 13.8% of all deaths among children aged 1 to 4 in 1985, and 26% of all deaths among children aged 5 to 14[8] (Figure 11).

Data Sources

State and Local

The local police department gathers data on motor vehicle fatalities and reports the data to the Fatal Accident Reporting System (FARS), coordinated by NHTSA. The agency responsible for compiling FARS data varies from state to state. The state department of transportation, state depart-

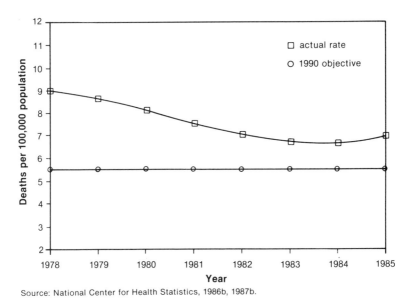

Source: National Center for Health Statistics, 1986b, 1987b.

Figure 11. Rates of motor vehicle accident fatalities for children ages 1 to 14, 1978–85 and 1990 Objective.

ment of motor vehicles, or state police may have this responsibility.

The registrar of vital statistics, usually located within the state or local health department, also maintains data on incidence and fatality rates based on death certificate reports. Each state also has a Governor's Highway Safety Commission, which can be a useful source of information on highway safety problems and programs, including legislation on the use of auto safety restraints and penalties for drinking drivers. Additionally, some states, such as Maryland and Massachusetts, have established systems for collecting population-based data on mortality and morbidity in childhood.

National

Two data sources provide detailed national information on traffic fatalities: the NCHS mortality file and the NHTSA FARS program. These sources agree closely on the total number of deaths.

NCHS publishes data on the incidence and rates of motor vehicle accident fatalities for children and youths in *Vital Statistics of the United States, Vol. II, Mortality*. Based on death certificate information reported through the VSRS, data are provided by sex, race, age group, and relationship of child or youth to vehicle (pedestrian, cyclist, passenger, or driver). There is approximately a three-year lag between the end of a calendar year and publication of data for that year.

More timely (two- to three-year lag) but less complete data are published in the *Advance Report of Final Mortality Statistics,* part of the Monthly Vital Statistics Report series. The *Advance Report* includes data on deaths and death rates from motor vehicle accidents by specified age group.

FARS is based on data collected continuously by police departments on the local level. Information is compiled at the state level and is reported to NHTSA, which publishes monthly fact sheets and quarterly and annual *FARS Reports.* General characteristics of each accident, people involved, relationship of child or youth to the vehicle, vehicles involved and related causes (such as car defects and blood-alcohol level of drivers) are all included. Data are reported by single-year ages and are available on a continuous basis, with a two- to three-month time lag between collection of data and publication of statistics.

Two additional sources of national data are the National Safety Council (NSC) and the Insurance Institute for Highway Safety (IIHS), both private organizations. The NSC's annual publication *Accident Facts* compiles data gathered by NCHS and NHTSA, plus data sent directly to NSC by 49 participating states. The IIHS periodically produces or supports research on the effect of policies and programs aimed at reducing motor vehicle fatalities.

The best national estimates of the incidence of nonfatal motor vehicle accidents are based on samples. NCHS's National Health Interview Survey provides limited information on motor vehicle crash injuries, which are a subset of a continuing national sample of health conditions. NHTSA's National Accident Sampling System data file contains information on nonfatal accidents from a stratified sample of police-reported crashes in 30 geographic areas.

Data Needs

National

There is a two- to three-year lag between the end of a calendar year and publication of final NCHS data for that year. This long lag makes it difficult to use timely data for purposes of planning and evaluating public policies and programs. NSC fatality data are partially based on NCHS vital statistics and are, therefore, subject to a similar time lag. Although FARS data are more timely, they are not available by race.

Although NCHS and NHTSA data closely agree on the total number of motor vehicle fatalities, these data systems are not linked, so gaps in knowledge of motor vehicle accidents remain. Numerous agencies are concerned with traffic accidents—the police, health services, insurance companies, local organizations, and various administrative bodies—but there is inadequate cooperation among them. The data available to each organization concerned, although incomplete, are complementary to the data available to other organizations. The police may have very detailed knowledge of the circumstances leading up to accidents, but see only the immediate consequences, whereas health services, which have the ability to assess longer term consequences, have limited knowledge of the precipitating circumstances.[3] Additionally, hospital-based research reveals significant underreporting of nonfatal injuries in most official statistics.

In addition to the gaps between information systems, there remains a discrepancy between what is already known about the cause and prevention of motor vehicle accident fatalities and the application of that knowledge. Despite technological progress in making automobiles more crash-worthy, lifesaving features have not been universally incorporated into cars produced for the public.

Also, little emphasis has been placed on the relationship between high-risk groups and effective means of protecting them. These relationships must be taken into account in planning effective approaches (especially measures that do not require individual attention and frequent effort) to reduce motor vehicle accident fatalities.

References

1. Baker S, O'Neill B, Karpf R. The injury fact book. Lexington, MA: Lexington Books, 1984.

2. Centers for Disease Control. Blood alcohol concentrations among young drivers—United States, 1982. MMWR 1983;32(16 Dec):646–8.

3. Deschamps J. Statistical data on traffic accidents in childhood. In: Prevention of traffic accidents in childhood. Copenhagen: World Health Organization, 1981.

4. DuMouchel W, Williams A, Zador P. Raising the alcohol purchase age: its effect on fatal motor vehicle crashes in 26 states. J Legal Studies (in press).

5. Haaga J. Children's seatbelt usage: evidence from the National Health Interview Survey. Am J Public Health 1986;76(Dec):1425–7.

6. Haddon W, Blumenthal M. Foreword. In: Ross H, ed. Deterring the drinking driver: legal policy and social control. Lexington, MA: Lexington Books, 1981.

7. National Center for Health Statistics. Current estimates from the National Health Interview Survey: United States. 1986. Vital and Health Statistics 10(160). DHHS Pub. No. (PHS)86–1588. Washington, DC: NCHS, 1986.

8. National Center for Health Statistics. Health—United States and prevention profile, 1986. DHHS Pub. No. (PHS)87–1232. Washington, DC: NCHS, 1986.

9. National Center for Health Statistics. Advance report of final mortality statistics, 1985. Monthly Vital Statistics Report 36(Aug). Supplement. DHHS Pub. No. (PHS)87–1120. Washington, DC: NCHS, 1987.

10. National Center for Health Statistics. Table 292. deaths for 282 selected causes by five-year age groups, color and sex, United States, 1979–85. Unpublished data. 1987.

11. National Center for Health Statistics. Table 292-A. death rates for 282 selected causes by five-year age groups, color and sex: United States, 1979–1985. Unpublished data. 1987.

12. National Highway Traffic Safety Administration. Effectiveness and efficiency of safety belt and child restraint usage programs. DOT Pub. No. (HS) 806–142. Washington, DC: DOT, 1982.

13. National Highway Traffic Safety Administration. Fatal Accident Reporting System, 1985. DOT Pub. No. (HS) 806–566. Washington, DC: DOT, 1987.

14. National Highway Traffic Safety Administration. 1986 traffic fatalities preliminary reports. DOT Pub. No. (HS) 807–097. Washington, DC: DOT, 1987.

15. National Safety Council. Accident facts, 1987 edition. Chicago: National Safety Council, 1987.

16. Public Health Service. Promoting health/preventing disease: objectives for the nation. DHHS Pub. No. (OM)81–0007. Washington, DC: PHS, 1980.

17. Sewell C, Hull H, Fenner J, Graff H, Pine J. Child restraint law effects on motor vehicle accident fatalities and injuries: the New Mexico experience. Pediatrics 1986;78:1079–84.

18. Wagenaar A, Webster D. Preventing injuries to children through compulsory automobile safety seat use. Pediatrics 1986;78:662–72.

19. Williams A. Fatal motor vehicle crashes involving teenagers. Pediatrician 1985;12: 37–40.

20. Williams A, Lund A. Seat belt use laws and occupant crash protection in the United States. Am J Public Health 1986;76(12):1438–42.

21. Williams A, Weeks J, Lund A. Voluntary seat belt use among high school students. Accident Analysis and Prevention 1983;15:161–5.

CHAPTER 5

Indicators Important to Infants, Children, and Youths of All Ages

Iron Deficiency Anemia

Definition

Iron deficiency is a pathologic condition in which there is an abnormally low concentration of hemoglobin, the iron-carrying component of red cells, in the blood. Iron deficiency can be caused by inadequate dietary intake of iron, low iron stores at birth, or blood loss.

Clinically, the two most frequently used screening tests for anemia are hematocrit (HCT), a measure of the proportion of blood that is composed of red cells, and hemoglobin (Hgb), a measure of the number of grams of hemoglobin in 100 ml of blood.

Indicators

- The percentage of children and youths within a population group who are at or below traditional cutoffs for low Hgb or HCT values for age and sex (see Table 11).
- The percentage of children and youths within a population group who have Hgb or HCT values below the 5th percentile for the U.S. population for age and sex (see Table 12).

Most health programs use only Hgb or HCT to screen children for nutritional anemia; hence, these measures are used to define this indicator. However, an expert scientific working group established to assess the biology of iron in the U.S. population concluded that a more sensitive means for identifying impaired iron status would use the following measures, with low values in any two indicating impaired iron status: transferrin saturation, erythrocyte protoporphyrin, and mean corpuscular volume. Routine addition of these tests on a clinical level would allow more comprehensive screening and better early detection of compromised iron status.[14]

Table 11. Traditional cutoff values for low hemoglobin and low hematocrit by age and sex.

Age	Sex	Lab value	
		Hgb (g/100 ml)	HCT (% rbc's)
6–23 mo	Female/Male	<10	<31
2–5 yr	Female/Male	<11	<34
6–14 yr	Female/Male	<12	<37
≥15 yr	Female	<12	<37
	Male	<13	<40

Source: CDC, 1985.

Table 12. Hemoglobin and hematocrit cutoff values based on the 5th percentile for children ages 6 months to 17 years by age and sex: United States, 1976–80.

Age	Sex	Lab value	
		Hgb (g/100 ml)	HCT (% rbc's)
6 mo–2 yr	Female	<10.5	<31.5
	Male	<10.4	<31.0
3–5 yr	Female	<11.0	<32.5
	Male	<11.0	<32.5
6–8 yr	Female	<11.3	<33.6
	Male	<11.3	<33.5
9–11 yr	Female	<11.6	<34.2
	Male	<11.6	<34.5
12–14 yr	Female	<11.7	<34.5
	Male	<12.1	<35.5
15–17 yr	Female	<11.4	<34.2
	Male	<12.9	<38.2

Source: Fulwood et al. 1982.

Note: New recommended reference criteria for anemia will be published shortly by CDC in *MMWR*. For further information, contact Faye Wong, Division of Nutrition, CDC, Atlanta.

Significance

Health Implications

The child with iron deficiency anemia may suffer from listlessness and fatigue, headache, or dizziness. Long-term, chronic anemia can lead to poor growth and weight gain, mental and physical sluggishness, palpitations and enlargement of the heart, impaired immune response, and a general inability to carry out the activities of childhood, including maintaining adequate school performance.[7, 11, 12, 17]

Policy and Program Implications

Iron deficiency anemia due to insufficient dietary intake is an indicator of the nutritional status of a population. It is both preventable and treatable, given an adequate diet, dietary supplements, or both. The proportion of infants, children, youths, and pregnant women with iron deficiency anemia reflects the adequacy and availability of food programs, prenatal services, well-baby care, and general preventive pediatric screening and care for a population.

Racial differences in HCT and Hgb levels have been widely reported in the literature, with blacks showing consistently lower values than whites of comparable age and sex. There is a good deal of controversy regarding the extent to which these differences can be attributed to genetic rather than to nutritional or socioeconomic factors, and the extent to which lower HCT and Hgb levels might be normal and healthy among blacks. Some researchers have suggested establishing separate standards for blacks; however, others note that most studies to date do not adequately control for socioeconomic status and that further study is necessary to determine the effect of lower HCT and Hgb values on the health status of blacks.[8, 10, 20]

Status and Trends

National

• Pediatric anemia, which in the vast majority of cases is iron deficiency anemia, is one of the most common nutritional problems in the United States. Particularly vulnerable are infants, preschoolers, and adolescents.[7, 9, 23]

• Data from the National Health and Nutrition Examination Survey of 1976–80 (NHANES II) indicate that poor children have consistently lower mean HCT and Hgb values than do nonpoor children. Among poor children ages 3 through 17, age-adjusted Hgb values were 13.1 for males and 12.7 for females compared with values of 13.5 for males and 13.1 for females among nonpoor children in the same age group. HCT values for poor children ages 3 through 17 were 38.6 for males and 37.4 for females, compared with 39.3 and 38.2, respectively, for nonpoor males and females ages 3 through 17.[9]

• Further analysis of NHANES II data (1976–80) indicates that infants from poor families are three times more likely than their nonpoor counterparts to be iron deficient.[6]

• Data from NHANES II (1976–80) indicate that mean HCT and Hgb values are consistently lower for black children in the United States than for white children. Among preschool children ages 3 through 5, for example, the mean Hgb values for boys are 11.9 for blacks and 12.4 for whites. Among girls ages 12 through 14, mean HCT values are 37.5 for blacks and 39.0 for whites. And among 15- through 17-year-old males, the mean HCT values are 41.9 for blacks and 43.0 for whites.[9]

• Data from the 1986 Pediatric Nutrition Surveillance System (PedNSS) indicate that among low-income children through age 17 monitored by CDC, 6.9% fell below the 5th percentile for HCT or Hgb. Blacks were most likely to be anemic, with 9.3% falling below the 5th percentile for HCT and 7.0% falling below the 5th percentile for Hgb. Hispanic children ranked second in risk of anemia; the percentage falling below the 5th percentile was 7.3% for HCT and 4.4% for Hgb.[4, 5]

• Among low-income children monitored by CDC in 1986, the age group most likely to have low HCT levels was 3- through 5-year-olds, with 13.2% of blacks; 9.4% of Hispanics; 7.4% of whites; 5.8% of Asian, Pacific Islander, and Southeast Asian refugees; and 5.7% of American Indians (Native Americans) falling below the 5th percentile. The age group most likely to have low Hgb values was 13- through 17-year-olds, with 17.4% of blacks; 12.8% of Hispanics; 11.9% of Asian, Pacific Islander, and Southeast Asian refugees; and 10.1% of whites falling below the 5th percentile (data on American Indians and Alaskan natives were unreliable for this age category).[5]

• Based on a review of data from six states consistently enrolled in the PedNSS, the CDC reports a 60% decline between 1975 and 1985 in the prevalence of anemia among low-income children under age six enrolled in public nutrition and health programs. The prevalence of anemia was significantly lower at follow-up visits than at initial visits; however, prevalences at both kinds of visits declined over the decade. CDC analysts conclude that the decline in anemia at initial visits reflects a general improvement in iron intake during infancy and early childhood, independent of participation in a program. However, the even lower prevalence at follow-up visits indicates that WIC and other public programs contribute to the reduction in anemia among high-risk populations.[3, 24]

State and Local

• A study of predominantly white, middle-class children in Minneapolis indicates a consistent decline in anemia over nearly two decades. Among children nine months to six years of age, seen at a private pediatric clinic, the rate of anemia decreased from 6.2% for the years 1969 through 1973 to 2.7% for the years 1982 through 1986. The researchers attribute this decline to an improved iron intake among infants and young children. Better iron intake is related to increased and prolonged use of breast-feeding, substitution of iron-fortified formula for cow's milk and unfortified formulas, use of iron-fortified infant cereals, and a generally heightened awareness among parents regarding the importance of iron in the diet.[25]

• Researchers in Memphis report dramatic declines in the frequency of low Hgb values among preschoolers living in high-poverty areas of the city. In 1977, 28% of tested children fell below the 3rd percentile for Hgb, compared with 12% in 1983. Despite this sizeable reduction, children from the poorest communities within Memphis run four times the predicted risk of low Hgb based on national norms.[26]

• In Minneapolis, the health department reports that 20% of low-income mothers and children in that city were found to be anemic in 1983—four times the rate in the general population. Among pregnant women studied, 33% were found to be anemic.[15]

• Data from the Maryland State Health Department for 1983 reveal that among children 18 to 24 months old, 14% of blacks and 11% of whites had anemia, and an additional 17% and 20%, respectively, had suspicious or borderline values. Additionally, approximately 9% of all children seen in Baltimore City's local health department clinics had a positive or borderline finding for anemia.[13]

• In Ramsey County, MN (St. Paul area), a study of low-income children under age seven revealed that 4% to 7% were anemic in 1983 (4.3% had low Hgb levels and 6.9% had low HCT levels). When data were analyzed by WIC status, 6.2% of WIC participants versus 12.6% of children eligible for but not enrolled in WIC had low HCT values. For Hgb values, 2.9% of WIC participants versus 4.6% of eligible nonparticipants had values below the cutoff for anemia.[1]

• In a study of the impact of the WIC program in Minneapolis, iron status was compared for two groups: toddlers participating in the WIC program in 1977 and low-income toddlers in the pre-WIC years of 1973 and 1974. For toddlers aged 12 through 17 months, 3.0% of WIC participants versus 14.1% of pre-WIC, low-income toddlers were anemic, and among 18- through 23-month-olds, 1.9% versus 6.4%, respectively, were anemic.[16]

Risk Factors

Minority children and children from families of low socioeconomic status are at increased risk of being iron deficient. Children in their preschool and adolescent years are also at increased risk for anemia.

U.S. Objective for Reducing Iron Deficiency Anemia

There are no national objectives established for reducing iron deficiency anemia among infants and children; however, in 1980, the U.S. Department of Health and Human Services established the following national objective for reducing iron deficiency anemia among pregnant women:

- By 1990, the proportion of pregnant women with iron deficiency anemia (as estimated by Hgb concentrations early in pregnancy) should be reduced to 3.5%. [In 1978, the proportion was 7.7%.][21]

Data Sources

State and Local

On the state level, the nutrition division of the state department of health may be able to provide population-based data on iron status. Some states conduct their own nutrition surveys using a random sample of the population. States participating in CDC's PedNSS may be able to provide data from "samples of convenience" on high-risk populations.

On the local level, the city or county health department and the local WIC, EPSDT (Early Periodic Screening, Diagnosis, and Treatment), and Head Start programs may be able to provide data. Agencies participating in the PedNSS should have quarterly and annual printouts analyzing HCT and Hgb values of clients by age, sex, and racial or ethnic group. Even if they are not part of the national program, some local programs such as WIC and EPSDT may compile data as part of their own reporting requirements. Although data from these programs cannot be used to generalize to an entire city or county population, they may be useful for looking at trends among selected populations.

A final source of local data may be pediatrics departments of local hospitals. In recent years, local hospitals in large cities (e.g., New York City, Boston, and Chicago) have conducted special nutritional studies of their pediatric emergency room populations.

National

The National Center for Health Statistics (NCHS) publishes the most current information on U.S. mean values and selected percentiles for HCT and Hgb by age, race (black and white), and poverty status in Vital and Health Statistics, Series 11. The most recent Series 11 report is based on data from NHANES II (1976–80).[9] The next Series 11 report will cover data from the Hispanic population in the United States (Hispanic HANES, 1982–84) and is scheduled for publication in 1989.

Extensive data on selected high-risk pediatric populations in the United States are published in *Nutrition Surveillance*, a periodic report from the PedNSS. The CDC surveillance system currently receives reports from health departments in 36 states, Puerto Rico, and the District of Columbia. These reports are based primarily on data from local WIC, EPSDT, Head Start, and Maternal and Child Health programs. *Nutrition Surveillance* includes data on the percentage of children (in participating programs) who fall below traditional cutoffs by age and sex for Hgb and HCT and the percentage who fall below the 5th percentile by age and sex for the United States as a whole. These data are provided by age group (6–11 months, 12–23 months, 2–5 years, and 6–9 years) and ethnic origin (white, black, Hispanic, Native American, and Asian). Five-year trend data on the percentage below traditional cutoffs are also available. The most recent *Nutrition Surveillance* dates from 1985 and covers 1983 data.[2]

More limited, but more timely reports from the PedNSS are published periodically in selected issues of *Morbidity and Mortality Weekly Report*. On a quarterly and annual basis, CDC also compiles PedNSS data from all participating states, including data on low HCT and Hgb; however, these data are not published or a widely distributed as *Nutrition Surveillance*.

CDC surveillance data on the percentage of children below the 5th percentile are based on special calculations using six-month age intervals, which give more accurate estimates than would be obtained using broader age categories. Based on these calculations, the proportion of children below the 5th percentile is consistently lower than the proportion below traditional cutoffs for low HCT and Hgb values. Analysts comparing data sets (trend data or local vs. national data) should exercise care to make sure that the same criteria are used for cutoffs and that calculations are based on the same age intervals.

Because CDC's surveillance information is not taken from a random or representative sample of the population, the sample is referred to as a "sample of convenience," and the data should be interpreted with caution. The PedNSS cannot be used to draw conclusions about the nutritional status of an entire community or of an entire at-risk population within the community. However, CDC notes that such samples of convenience can be used to determine the prevalence of nutritional problems among participating children and to evaluate the effectiveness of clinical services to these children. A more detailed description of the surveillance program and its uses is available in the CDC paper *Surveillance of Nutritional Status in the United States*.[22]

Older, but still useful background data on iron status of children are available from the first two major national nutritional surveys, both conducted in 1968 through 1970: the Ten-State Nutrition Survey (TSNS), which focused on low-income populations in 10 states plus New York City, and the Preschool Nutrition Survey (PNS), which looked at a random sample of U.S. children ages one through five. Reports from the TSNS are available from the Nutrition Division of CDC. The PNS data are available as a supplement to *Pediatrics,* published by the American Academy of Pediatrics.[18]

Data Needs

National

There are a number of significant gaps in national data systems to assess anemia among U.S. children. The NHANES provides population-based data, but these data are limited by infrequent collection and reporting cycles. Data collection for NHANES III began in September 1988 and continue over a six-year period. Midpoint data covering the first three years will first be available on public-use data tapes in 1992, with publishing scheduled for 1993. With 10- to 12-year intervals between studies, NHANES cannot possibly keep an adequate pulse on the nutritional status of the nation's children.

Analysis and reporting of NHANES II data for HCT and Hgb are extremely limited. Although data are collected for vulnerable subpopulations (defined by age, race, and poverty status), there is no attempt to report by subpopulation the percentage of children who fall either below traditional cutoffs for HCT or Hgb values or below the 5th percentile for the population as a whole. In addition, poverty status data are published only for very broad age categories, such as 3- through 17-year-olds.

PedNSS data are limited because they are based on a sample of convenience. The data do not necessarily reflect the nutritional status of all low-income children in the United States, but rather the status of children participating in certain programs in certain states.

Reporting of annual data in *Nutrition Surveillance* has been delayed for several years, with the most recent publication covering 1983 data. It is anticipated that the report covering 1984 data will be published in 1989. In part, this delay has allowed CDC to make composite and individual state data available to participating states on a quarterly and annual basis; however, these data are not published, nor are they as widely distributed as *Nutrition Surveillance*. Resumed publication of *Nutrition Surveillance* should make CDC's valuable data and analysis more accessible to a wide range of users.

References

1. Brown J, Serdula M, Cairns K, Godes J, Jacobs D, Elmer P. Ethnic group differences in nutritional status of young children from low-income areas of an urban county. Am J Clin Nutr 1986;44:838–44.

2. Centers for Disease Control. Nutrition surveillance: annual summary 1983. DHHS Pub. No. (CDC)85-8295. Washington, DC: CDC, 1985.

3. Centers for Disease Control. Declining anemia prevalence among children enrolled in public nutrition and health programs—selected states, 1975–1985. MMWR 1986;35(36):565–6.

4. Centers for Disease Control. Table 6, CDC pediatric nutrition surveillance: clinics ranked by low hemoglobin and/or low hematocrit, reporting period 01/01/86 to 12/31/86. Unpublished table (26 Jun). Sequence No. 017858. Atlanta: 1987.

5. Centers for Disease Control. Table 10, pediatric nutrition surveillance: statewide summary of indicators by age and ethnic groups, reporting period 01/01/86 to 12/31/86. Unpublished table (26 Jun). Sequence No. 017869. Atlanta: 1987.

6. Dallman P. Has routine screening of infants for anemia become obsolete in the United States? Pediatrics 1987;80(Sep):439–40.

7. Dallman P, Siimes M, Stekel A. Iron deficiency in infancy and childhood. Am J Clin Nutr 1980;33(Jan):86–118.

8. Dutton D. Hematocrit levels and race: an argument against the adoption of separate standards in screening for anemia. Paper presented at the American Public Health Association meetings, 18 Oct 1978, Los Angeles.

9. Fulwood R, Johnson C, Bryner J, Gunter E, McGrath C. Hematological and nutritional biochemistry reference data for persons 6 months–74 years of age: United States, 1976–1980. Vital and Health Statistics, Series 11, No. 232. DHHS Pub. No. (PHS)83-1682. Washington, DC: National Center for Health Statistics, 1982.

10. Garn S, Smith N, Clark D. The magnitude and the implications of apparent race differences in hemoglobin values. Letter to the Editor. Am J Clin Nutr 1975;28(Jun):563–8.

11. Good R, Hanson L, Edelman R. Infections and undernutrition. Nutr Rev 1982;40(Apr):119–28.

12. Goodhart R, Shils M, eds. Modern nutrition in health and disease. 6th ed. Philadelphia: Lea & Febiger, 1980.

13. Governor's Task Force on Food and Nutrition. Interim Report. Annapolis, MD: State of Maryland, 1984.

14. Joint Nutrition Monitoring Evaluation Committee. Nutrition monitoring in the United States: a progress report from the Joint Nutrition Monitoring Evaluation Committee. DHHS Pub. No. 86-1255. Washington, DC: U.S. Department of Health and Human Services and U.S. Department of Agriculture, 1986.

15. Milhous P. Testimony before Committee on Labor and Human Resources, Field Investigation on Hunger in America, U.S. Senate, 19 Nov 1983. Minneapolis Health Department. Minneapolis, MN.

16. Miller V, Swaney S, Deinard A. Impact of the WIC program on the iron status of infants. Pediatrics 1985;75(Jan):100–5.

17. Oski F. The nonhematologic manifestations of iron deficiency. Am J Dis Child 1979;133(Mar):315–22.

18. Owen G, Kram K, Garry P, Lowe J, Lubin A. A study of nutritional status of preschool children in the United States, 1968–1970. Pediatrics, Supplement–Part II 1974;53(4):597–646.

19. Pollitt E, Leibel R. Iron deficiency and behavior. J Pediatr 1976;88(Mar):372–81.

20. Popkin B, Akin J, Kaufman M, MacDonald M. Nutritional program options for maternal and child health. In: Better health for our children: a national strategy; vol 4, Report of the Select Panel for the Promotion of Child Health. Washington, DC: PHS, 1981;87–125.

21. Public Health Service. Promoting health/preventing disease: objectives for the nation. DHHS Pub. No. (OM)81-0007. Washington, DC: PHS, 1980.

22. Robbins G. Surveillance of nutritional status in the United States. Mimeographed paper. Atlanta: Centers for Disease Control, 1980.

23. Starfield B. Iron deficiency Anemia. In: Children's medical care needs and treatments: report of the Harvard Child Health Project. Cambridge, MA: Ballinger, 1977: 77–120.

24. Yip R, Binkin N, Fleshood L, Trowbridge F. Declining prevalence of anemia among low-income children in the United States. JAMA 1987;258(25 Sep):1619–23.

25. Yip R, Walsh K, Goldfarb M, Binkin N. Declining prevalence of anemia in childhood in a middle-class setting: a pediatric success story? Pediatrics 1987;80(3 Sep):330–4.

26. Zee P, DeLeon M, Roberson P, Chen C. Nutritional improvement of poor urban preschool children: a 1983-1987 comparison. JAMA 1985;253(14 Jun):3269–72.

Child Abuse and Neglect

Definition

The term child abuse and neglect does not encompass one problem, or even two, but a multitude of problems that can occur in the day-to-day interactions between children and the adults responsible for their care. Based on the definition used by the National Center on Child Abuse and Neglect (NCCAN), a case of child abuse or neglect is one in which, through intentional acts, a parent, guardian, or other adult caretaker causes foreseeable and avoidable injury or impairment to a child under age 18 years or contributes to the unreasonable prolongation or worsening of an existing injury or impairment in a child under age 18 years.[20]

Indicators

- The number of deaths from child abuse or neglect within a defined population.
- The number of confirmed cases of child abuse or neglect reported by an established surveillance team or project for a specific geographic area.

Significance

Implications for Health and Social Functioning

Child abuse or neglect may result in severe and permanent physical disfigurement, disability, or death caused by burns, lacerations, fractures, contusions, hemorrhages, venereal disease, malnourishment, or untreated injury or disease.[46] Children who survive physical assaults or neglect may suffer profound psychosocial disturbances. Although not yet conclusive, research now suggests that maltreated children may be at increased risk of becoming delinquents or runaways, of exhibiting learning disabilities or behavioral problems, of becoming criminals as adults, and of mistreating their own children.[15, 18, 27, 29]

Policy and Program Implications

Deaths from and confirmed cases of child abuse and neglect represent breakdowns in the ability of family units to protect, nurture, and support children. These adverse outcomes reflect the need for a wide range of well-coordinated preventive measures that reduce the risk from specific individual, family, and social conditions associated with maltreatment. Needed services include perinatal support and parent education programs to prepare parents for the tasks ahead and to help parents establish realistic expectations for child development; early, regular screening and treatment programs for children, to detect and promptly address developmental problems; self-help support groups for abusing and neglecting parents to help them cope with guilt and social isolation; programs for abused and neglected children to minimize the physical, social, and psychological consequences of their maltreatment; family support services, such as crisis lines; health services, including family planning; day care, child care, and marriage counseling; respite centers; and community development activities that increase employment opportunities, improve low-income housing, and increase access to job training.[11, 12, 14]

Status and Trends

National

• An estimated 1000 children in the United States die from abuse or neglect each year.[21] In the 29 states reporting fatality information to the Select Committee on Children, Youth and Families, 587 children died from abuse or neglect in 1985.[24] Preliminary findings from a survey by the National Committee for the Prevention of Child Abuse indicate that deaths from child abuse increased in 1986.[25]

• The number of reported cases of child abuse and neglect has increased 180% in the United States over the past nine years. In 1976, the first year reports were available, 669,000 children were reported as maltreated.[3] By 1985, the number of children reported as abused or neglected reached nearly 1.9 million (Figure 12).[24]

• Physical abuse is the type of maltreatment most commonly linked to fatality; however, the majority of reports indicate neglect is the most common form of maltreatment, involved in three out of every five reported cases in 1985.[2, 24]

• Reports of sexual abuse of children increased dramatically between 1983 and 1984. In 1983, 8.5% of reported cases of child abuse and neglect involved sexual abuse. In 1984, this figure was up to 13.3%—an increase of 56% over the previous year. This increase in the proportion of cases translates into an increase of 35% in the estimated number of U.S. children who were reported as sexually abused.[2, 7]

• Sexual abuse of children may be more prevalent than official reports suggest. Retrospective studies of adults indicate that 1 in 4 girls and 1 in

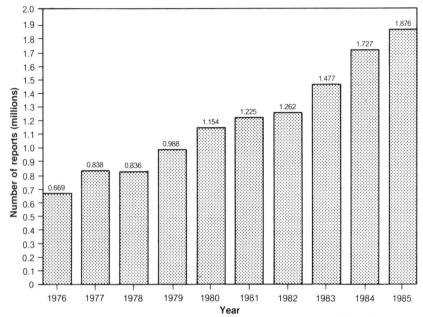

(Data for 1985 do not include Puerto Rico, the U.S. Virgin Islands, Guam, and the Marianas.)
Source: Select Committee on Children, Youth and Families, 1987b.

Figure 12. Number of reports of child abuse and neglect, 1976–85.

10 boys were sexually abused at some point during childhood or adolescence.[10] A study of 1200 college-age women found that although 28% had sexual experience with an adult before age 13, only 6% of the incidents had been reported.[19]

• The types of maltreatment reported vary by age and sex. In 1985, the average age of involved children was 7.1 years.[3] In general, neglect is most common among young children and appears to occur less often among older children, whereas sexual and emotional maltreatment occur least often among young children and become more common as children age. The highest rates of physical abuse are found among the oldest children.[23]

• Most studies find no significant differences between the proportion of males and females reported as abused and neglected. Nonetheless, girls are more likely to be abused, and boys are more likely to be neglected, with the gender difference becoming more pronounced with increasing age.[21]

• A racial breakdown indicates that of the children reported to have been maltreated in the United States in 1984, 67% were white, 21% were black, and 10% were Hispanic. These proportions have remained relatively stable over time.[2]

• A strong relationship exists between family income and recognized maltreatment, with children from low-income families more likely than those from higher income families to be recognized as maltreated.[11, 21]

• The extent to which recognized maltreatment reflects true incidence is unknown; however, recent research suggests that abuse in high-income white families may be disproportionately underreported by professionals, reflecting both race and class bias.[13]

State and Local

• With the exception of Wyoming, every state reported an increase in the number of cases of child abuse and neglect between 1981 and 1985.[24]

• Alabama, Arizona, Illinois, Kansas, North Dakota, Texas, and Utah noted a trend toward more serious cases of child maltreatment. Connecticut, Hawaii, Pennsylvania, and West Virginia have witnessed increases in the number of seriously physically abused children.[24]

• In 1985, Maine, Nevada, and North Carolina indicated that cases have become more complex in the past nine years. The District of Columbia, Illinois, Kentucky, Rhode Island, and Wyoming have had increases in the frequency of family dysfunction.[24]

• Many states and localities have noted an association between unemployment and child abuse. For example, over the past 17 years, the incidence of cases of physical abuse in Denver rose and fell with the unemployment rate in Colorado.[25] Between 1980 and 1981, the unemployment rate in Detroit rose from 15% to 17%. During this same period, the number of substantiated child abuse and neglect cases rose 37%. In Wisconsin, cases of child abuse increased by 6% in 1981; however, in the 10 counties with the greatest rise in unemployment, the number of reported cases rose by 123%. It appears, also, that high unemployment rates may be associated with increases in the severity of maltreatment. In Texas, a state that has been hard hit economically, the number of life-threatening cases increased by 30% over a one-year period.[8]

Risk Factors

A review of the literature indicates that certain characteristics of the child, the family unit, and the socioeconomic environment put a child at increased risk of abuse or neglect.

Risk factors that are characteristics of the child include being born prematurely or being low birth weight;[5,17] being a "graduate" of a neonatal intensive care unit; and having serious defects, disabilities, or chronic illness.[18,30]

Family unit factors include alcoholic parent(s); absence of either the natural mother or the natural father from the home; an unusually high level of stress in the family; violence between parents; a parent with a history of being abused as a child; and a parent who is extremely immature, or who has unrealistically high expectations of the child.[9,16]

Socioeconomic factors include the absence of adequate social support systems for individual family members or the family unit (e.g., being isolated from supportive religious or social groups); living in poverty or with unemployment (especially recent unemployment); living in low-quality or inadequate housing; and living in a high-crime area or an area with a very transient population—both factors that increase stress.[1,8,11,21]

U.S. Objective for Reducing Child Abuse and Neglect

The U.S. Department of Health and Human Services set the following objective for reducing maltreatment of children:

- By 1990, injuries and deaths to children inflicted by abusing parents should be reduced by at least 25%. (Reliable baseline data were unavailable. At the time the objective was set, estimates varied from 200,000 to 4 million cases occurring each year in this country.)[22]

Action to prevent and reduce child abuse has been hampered by the lack of recent, reliable national data on the incidence and prevalence of the problem. Progress toward meeting this objective is therefore difficult to measure, and the likelihood of achieving the goal by 1990 is unknown.[26]

Efforts to prevent or reduce child abuse and neglect have been hindered further by decreases in federal funding. The Child Abuse Prevention and Treatment Act (CAPTA) funds are devoted solely to the prevention, identification, and treatment of child abuse, but Title XX of the Social Services Block Grant remains the largest source of federal funds available to states for child welfare and child protective services. Both CAPTA and Title XX sustained funding cuts (30% and 21%, respectively) in FY 1981, the same year the U.S. objective to reduce child abuse was established. By FY 1985, modest funding increases had not restored funds to FY 1981 levels.[24]

Data Sources

State and Local

State and local data reflect reported cases of child maltreatment rather than true incidence. All 50 states plus the District of Columbia, American Samoa, Guam, Puerto Rico, and the Virgin Islands have enacted legislation mandating reporting of suspected child maltreatment to public agencies. Most of these jurisdictions have a central registry of reported cases, maintained by the division of child protective services (CPS). In California, the department of justice maintains registry data.

The CPS division of the city or county social services department is the agency responsible for cases of child maltreatment in most local areas. Data at the local level may prove the most useful for monitoring changes because the problem of variation in reporting, recording, and investigation practices should be minimized. The local surveillance team can provide information on the kinds of cases included in local data and on changes in reporting and investigation practices over time.

National

National data on child abuse and neglect are limited to cases and deaths reported to protective service agencies and other investigative agencies (police departments, public health departments, etc.) or known to professionals in schools, hospitals, and other major institutions. Because unreported cases are not included, and estimates of the extent of child abuse and neglect vary by source of information, the true incidence of child abuse and neglect is unknown.[2, 28]

Study Findings: National Study of the Incidence and Severity of Child Abuse and Neglect, published in 1981 by NCCAN,[21] provides estimates of the national incidence of child abuse and neglect. This report examines a national sample of cases and deaths reported in 26 counties. Data are reported by type of abuse or neglect; severity of the child's injury or impairment; sex, age, and ethnic group of the child; the type of county of residence (urban, rural, or suburban); and the source of the reports. In 1985, NCCAN funded a follow-up study of the incidence of child abuse and neglect. When available, the data will provide information on the effectiveness of efforts to detect, prevent, and reduce child maltreatment.

NCCAN also maintains a clearinghouse on child abuse and neglect. This clearinghouse provides the public with information on articles, studies, and reports on topics such as incidence, service programs, predictors, risk factors, outcomes, and court decisions.

Another source of national data is the American Association for Protecting Children (AAPC). A division of the American Humane Association, the AAPC since 1973 has assembled and analyzed information on cases and deaths reported to CPS agencies. *Highlights of Official Child Neglect and Abuse Reporting*, available for each year since 1976, contains case data from states and territories and information on the number of reported cases of child abuse and neglect. States and territories voluntarily participate in this system. Composite data are presented by the type of maltreatment; stress factors in the family; relationship of the child to the perpetrator; age, sex, and race of the child; the source and type of report; and the status of the case and services provided. There is approximately an 18-month lag between the end of a calendar year and publication of data for that year.

Data Needs

State and Local

There can be a wide variation in the adequacy of data reported to the state by local jurisdictions. Although statewide guidelines are established for reporting and follow-up, the local agencies implementing these programs may face staff and budget constraints that force them to become highly selective in choosing cases for and determining the extent of investigation. Any analysis of changes in the number of reported and substantiated cases should take into account variations in recording and reporting practices.

National

The most recent national estimates of the incidence and severity of child abuse and neglect are based on 1979–80 data. However, CAPTA, reauthorized in October 1984, provided funds for another two-year NCCAN study of the incidence and severity of child maltreatment. The report will be based on 1984–85 data.

Although the standardization and quality of state-operated information systems have improved in recent years, problems often emerge when state data are aggregated. For example, interpreting national statistics on the number of reports to CPS agencies is complicated by the fact that some states tabulate families but others count individual children.

Other definitional and procedural differences among states further complicate interpretation of state-collected data. Traditionally, child abuse or neglelct, like juvenile delinquency, marriage, or divorce, is litigated in the family court system and, therefore, left to individual states' discretion. Although most states have incorporated some of the provisions of the NCCAN Model Act, there is no mandate for uniform reporting definitions and procedures.

National summaries based on reporting from sources other than CPS agencies (police departments, hospitals, etc.) are subject to inaccuracies and inconsistencies due to jurisdictional differences in accuracy of detection, public and professional awareness, degree of enforcement, reporting bias, and sampling techniques.

The AAPC collects information on child abuse and neglect only at the time a report is filed; hence, data on fatalities are underreported as fatalities are tabulated only if cited on initial case reports. No system for follow-up, which is essential for information on fatalities, is built into this data base.

Through 1984, the AAPC collected and analyzed data from all 50 states, the District of Columbia, Puerto Rico, the Virgin Islands, Guam, and the Marianas. However, because of funding constraints, AAPC's analysis of 1985 data is restricted to 5 states, thus limiting both the scope of the information and the usefulness of the data for comparisons over time.

A complete picture of the extent and character of recognized child abuse and neglect in the United States cannot be achieved from current official statistics. States' disclosure of data to organizations maintaining national data bases, such as AAPC and NCCAN, is completely voluntary. The gap in standardized official data is exacerbated by this unevenness of reporting.

References

1. American Association for Protecting Children. Unemployment and child abuse and neglect reporting. Denver, CO: American Humane Association, 1983.

2. American Association for Protecting Children. Highlight of official child neglect and abuse reporting, 1984. Denver, CO: American Humane Association, 1986.

3. American Association for Protecting Children. Highlights of official child neglect and abuse reporting, 1985. Denver, CO: American Humane Association, 1987.

4. American Medical Association. AMA diagnostic and treatment guidelines concerning child abuse and neglect. Connecticut Medicine 1986;50(Feb):122–8.

5. Benedict M, White B. Selected perinatal factors and child abuse. Am J Public Health 1985;75(7):780–1.

6. Bergman A, Larsen R, Mueller B. Changing spectrum of serious child abuse. Pediatrics 1986;77(Jan):113–6.

7. Child Welfare League of America. Too young to run: the status of child abuse in America. Washington, DC: Child Welfare League of America, 1986.

8. Coolsen P. Unemployment and child abuse. Caring 1982;8(4):6–7,10.

9. Famularo R, Stone K, Barnum R, Whorton R. Alcoholism and severe child maltreatment. Am J Orthopsychiatr 1986;56(Jul):481–4.

10. Finkelhor D. Child sexual abuse. New York: Free Press, 1984.

11. Garbarino J. A preliminary study of some ecological correlates of child abuse: the impact of socioeconomic stress on mothers. Child Development 1976;47:178–85.

12. Gray E, DiLeonardi J. Evaluating child abuse prevention programs. Chicago: National Committee for Prevention of Child Abuse, 1982.

13. Hampton R, Newberger E. Child abuse incidence and reporting by hospitals: significance of severity, class, and race. Am J Public Health 1985;75(1):56–60.

14. Howze D, Kotch J. Role of stress and social support in the occurrence of child abuse and neglect. Chapel Hill, NC: University of North Carolina, 1982.

15. Lash T, Sigal H, Dudzinski D. State of the child: New York City II. New York: Foundation for Child Development, 1980.

16. Leventhal J. Risk factors for child abuse: methodologic standards in case-control studies. Pediatrics 1981;68(May):684–90.

17. Leventhal J, Berg A, Egerter S. Is intrauterine growth retardation a risk for child abuse? Pediatrics 1987;79(Apr):515–9.

18. Mullins J. The relationship between child abuse and handicapping conditions. J Schl Health 1986;56(Apr):134–6.

19. National Association of Social Workers. Child abuse in America. Washington, DC: National Association of Social Workers, 1984.

20. National Center on Child Abuse and Neglect. Model Child Protection Act with commentary, draft. Washington, DC: 1977.

21. National Center on Child Abuse and Neglect. Study findings: national study of the incidence and severity of child abuse and neglect. DHHS Pub. No. OHDS 81-30325. Washington, DC: 1981.

22. Public Health Service. Promoting health/preventing disease: objectives for the nation. DHHS Pub. No. (OM)81–0007. Washington, DC: PHS, 1980.

23. Russell A, Trainor C. Trends in child abuse and neglect: a national perspective. Denver, CO: American Humane Association, 1984.

24. Select Committee on Children, Youth and Families. Abused children in America: victims of official neglect. U.S. House of Representatives (31 Jul). Washington, DC: 1987.

25. Select Committee on Children, Youth and Families. Child abuse and neglect in America: the problem and the response. U.S. House of Representatives (3 Mar). Washington, DC: 1987.

26. Silverman M, Lalley T, Rosenberg M, Smith J, Parron D, Jacobs J. Control of stress and violent behavior: mid-course review of the 1990 Health Objectives. Public Health Reports 1988;103(Jan–Feb):39–49.

27. Smith C, Berkman D, Fraser W. A preliminary national assessment of child abuse and neglect and the juvenile justice system: the shadows of distress. NCJ No. 64969. Washington, DC: National Juvenile Justice Assessment Centers, U.S. Department of Justice, 1981.

28. Task Force on Family Violence. Data collection and reporting. Final report. Washington, DC: U.S. Department of Justice, 1984.

29. Vachss A. Child abuse: a ticking bomb. Change 1982;5(3):6.

30. White R, Benedict M, Wulff L, Kelley M. Physical disabilities as risk factors for child maltreatment. Am J Orthopsychiatr 1987;57(Jan):93–101.

CHAPTER 6

Health Policy for Children:
Where We Stand

A tide of evidence confirms that recent trends for the health of the maternal and child population are unfavorable. Participation in prenatal care, rates of low birth weight, and infant mortality rates have all slowed or worsened, especially for vulnerable population subgroups. Immunization rates for preschool children have declined and outbreaks of preventable infectious disease have increased. Insofar as falling immunization rates indicate a decline in well-child health visits, an increase in hard-to-measure preventable morbidity may be presumed. Well documented child abuse and neglect continue to increase, as do suicides, especially among young white males.

Teenage childbearing attracts justifiable attention, but the trends are not always interpreted accurately. Teenage fertility has declined steadily in recent years, continuing a trend that has endured over recent decades. Childbearing among older age groups has declined even faster. This circumstance, taken together with the increased number of teenagers from the 1950s baby boom, means a relatively high proportion of all infants are born to teenage parents. The need for services and supports specific to that population is clearly demonstrated.

Fatalities and injuries from motor vehicle accidents increase, associated with an increase in recreational driving, often in combination with substance abuse. Trends for non–motor vehicle accident fatalities for children have improved, suggesting that the adequacy of housing and toddler supervision have not worsened in aggregate even though homelessness increasingly involves children.

One of the few indicators to improve is the rate of iron deficiency anemia among poor children. Widespread fortification of foods, including infant formulas, with iron has helped solve the problem. The utility of data on iron deficiency anemia as a marker for general nutritional status may have been weakened.

Some indicators are notable for identifying the deterioration of data systems. Inadequate current data are available on growth stunting, lead poisoning, and immunization rates. Small area studies suggest that these problems continue to be widespread.

Introductory comments to this work emphasized that policy does not necessarily derive from data. In the context of the practice in the United States for evolving health policy out of the negotiations of competing interest groups, good data should elevate the level of argumentation, and an enlightened policy should emerge. The following discussion attempts to identify some of the considerations that shape health policy, and concludes with recommendations that are believed to be consistent with the

force of these issues and responsive to the health status trends documented in the preceding pages.

The Reagan Years

The nation's experience with health policy during the Reagan years has
clarified several troublesome issues and confounded others. Whether in
balance they open the way toward bold new actions to improve children's
health is by no means clear. A ferment grows, unmatched in more than
a decade, to expand children's entitlements to health care. Confounding
issues threaten to work, as they have in the past, to frustrate these efforts
and to perpetuate persistent neglects and inequities. Progress toward over-
coming barriers to new programs may be helped by examining some of
the separate elements of children's health policy at the close of the Reagan administration.

The central theme of Reagan policy, dubbed "New Federalism," was
initially advanced during the second Nixon administration and put into
place by the Omnibus Budget Reconciliation Act of 1981. The policy's
central theme holds that services are best generated and distributed in competitive economic markets, unfettered by government controls. A subtheme
proposes that, insofar as government retains a role to render services, those
functions should be pushed toward state and local levels.

Reagan policies not only reduced social entitlements but redistributed
the tax burden in order to accumulate wealth that presumably would be
used to fuel the nation's economic growth. Other changes included block
grants of federal funds to the states, which reduced the level of federal
financing for the merged programs, eliminated the protective priorities
that derive from categorical financing, increased the separate discretion
of the states to determine their levels of effort to continue many programs,
and eliminated the reporting procedures and data collection that had been
attached to many of them. The new policies sought to reduce the size and
influence of government—to get it "off our backs."

The new policies assumed that the origins of nineteenth century American
vigor emerged from the investments of a wealthy, privileged class, rather
than from the enterprise of an emerging middle class, newly enfranchised
as participants in distributive democracy and protected by a growing role
for government to safeguard against social neglect and against the abuses
of private interests. The great productivity of the United States derived
from releasing the latent energies and talents of a middle class that enjoyed improved health and bright personal prospects.[1] Pushing a growing
portion of the middle class into poverty and redistributing income in fa-

vor of the wealthy runs counter to the national interest in many ways, including sapping the health and vigor of the largest and most productive segment of the population.

The Reagan years did not bring about a reduction in the size of government; it continued to grow. Growth of social spending to develop human capital was greatly reduced; military spending was increased to unprecedented levels. Non-means-tested social benefit programs continued to grow, while means-tested programs were proportionately reduced, contributing, along with the reduction of taxes on high incomes, to a widening gap between rich and poor.

In 1982 unemployment rates rose to levels unprecedented since the Great Depression, followed by a slow return of favorable employment rates and improvement in some other economic indicators. The extent to which the economic recovery can be attributed to reinvestment of accumulated wealth rather than government's deficit spending is by no means clear. For example, some analysts suggest that concentrated wealth enabled corporate mergers and buy-outs that added little productive capacity to the economy and had the effect of reducing competition. What is abundantly clear is that the economic recovery did not reach children. Their parents' job shifts tended to result in reduced wages and without fringe benefits such as health insurance. The proportion of children living in poverty-level households rose dramatically in 1981 and has not come back down.

The Reagan years clarified certain issues related to health policy for children and blurred others.

Some Clarifications

The Roles of Different Levels of Government

A vacillating dynamic affecting the locus of responsibility between federal and state levels of government has troubled health policy for most of this century. Compromises written into the Social Security Act of 1935 established the ambiguity. Some programs (old age security, survivors' benefits, and disability insurance) were federalized; other programs (child welfare, vocational rehabilitation, and public health services) were left to the considerable discretion of the states for implementation and definition of benefits. The amendments of 1965 (Medicare and Medicaid) entrenched the inconsistency. Medicare emerged as national age-specific health insurance, inclusive of the entire population over age 65 without means testing. Medicaid, on the other hand, was implemented differently by each state with great variation in benefits, consistent largely in the ethic to exclude ineligible populations. Other health initiatives of the 1960s (Office of Economic Opportunity, and Special Projects of Title V for Maternal and Child Health) strengthened the federal role directly to provide services for neglected populations, essentially bypassing state and local public agencies, and possibly contributing to the weakness of their programs and initiatives.

The Reagan policies tended to minimize the federal role as provider of health services and to accentuate the federal role in financing health care, either by means of social insurance or by grants to the states. Although Reagan's fiscal policies placed an increased financial burden on state governments and on out-of-pocket payments, the federal role sharpened to a clearer emphasis as buyer of health care.

Insofar as governmentally sponsored health services are required, they are provided either directly by agencies of state and local government or under contract with them. That mission is growing. A recent Government Accounting Office survey revealed that 60% of poor pregnant women receive their prenatal care in public clinics, largely sponsored by health departments.[10]

A residual federal responsibility for sponsored services persists on behalf of migrant and Indian populations and of communities demonstrably underserved. Survival of this function illustrates a continuing need for a federal role as guarantor of health care for populations not otherwise served. Federal support of more than 500 community health centers confirms that the need is substantial.

Lowered Expectations from Market Competition

After eight years of shrinking entitlements and promotion of market approaches for delivery of health care, neither the quality/price dyad nor access has responded favorably. A leading economist analyzed present circumstances and concluded that competition never really happened.[5] Certainly, no one was competing to provide health care for the enlarged number of poverty-level children who were not protected by either public or private insurance.

Another leading economist, Enthoven, perceived by many people as an apostle of market approaches, reported that he had been misunderstood.[4] He now advocates *managed* competition, and then only in the context of *universal insurance coverage*. Regulatory management of medical care and universal insurance coverage are causes that have not been widely advocated since the mid-1970s, but interest in them grows. As with the recognition of Communist China, bold strokes with the taint of liberalism are sometimes most effectively promoted from conservative quarters.

The Need for Government to Participate

Private and voluntary components are predominant in American health care and show every promise of enduring, but structural changes since 1965 have been profound. Voices that deny a role for government to manage these changes in the consumer's interest have faded. Even the interests of physicians, once at the vanguard of resistance to government medicine, may be served alongside the consumer's interests by some governmental protection from corporate medical management.[9] The anticipated modes of governmental action leave room for argument, but few people deny that interventions are required beyond paying for whatever the medical system is selling. Private insurance companies, hospitals, health maintenance organizations, and office-based practitioners continue to serve most people; government pays an increasing part of the bill and is increasingly likely to regulate content of care through payment practices.

Relying on the Mainstream

The preamble to Medicaid presumed that economic barriers to medical care would be removed so that poor people could benefit from the same mainstream services that were enjoyed by financially secure populations. Even as the mainstream has been altered to incorporate capitation payments and managed care, the evidence is overwhelming that families suffering from socioeconomic hardship require something different from what the mainstream provides. Nutritional supplementation, counseling and education, case work, psychological evaluations, transportation, housing and environmental protection—these are all ingredients of successful interventions not often found in the mainstream. They are more commonly mobilized around comprehensive community organized health care programs, usually under public auspices or as demonstration projects enjoying temporary foundation support.

Practitioners' widespread denial of services to Medicaid recipients is often attributed to low levels of compensation and to "red tape." Those deterrents are real, but so is the frustration that attends efforts to cope with complex biosocial problems using only conventional office-based resources. Conventional medical care meets the needs of most people most of the time, but it is not sufficient for many of the most pressing health needs of children suffering from chronic or disabling disease and from various deprivations. Organized, comprehensive community programs are required. New laws requiring schools to provide health care for children with special needs beginning at birth stand as testimony to unmet need. The gap, however, is apt to continue, as few school districts have the expertise or resources to cope with these large responsibilities.

Some Confounding Issues

Health Care as a Right—Universal Approaches

Policy formulations that protect a presumed right to health care are not as conspicuous as they were 10 years ago. Extension of the principle of social insurance to include all children fights a weary battle against incrementalism that perpetuates a means-tested approach to benefits. The advocates for improved services for children have chosen the path of pushing Medicaid eligibilities up the income scale, accentuating the expensive and annoying screening procedures for certification. That course has been pursued not because it shows most promise, but because it seemed politically feasible. The outer limits of political feasibility for children's health may not have been fully explored.

Early experience with recent expansions of Medicaid benefits and eligibilities for pregnant women and young children is not encouraging. Funds that were previously earmarked for community-based preventive health services in maternal and child health have been diverted to help pay the hospital bills for newly eligible maternity patients. Hospitals rejoice that their problems of uncompensated care are reduced, but local health departments, struggling to provide prenatal care for uninsured women, despair that agency funds have been cut in the face of a larger eligible population. Medicaid reimbursements for these women are not making up the difference.

Medicaid expansion is increasing the utilization of prenatal care in local health departments, but progress is slow. Certification review for a new client requires 2 ½ hours in at least one state (North Carolina), much more than the time required for a thorough prenatal visit. Conscientious certification examiners can process only two or three new clients per day. The process, which aims to maximize exclusion, is so thorough that only the most committed pregnant women will subject themselves to it. Why go through the ordeal of producing rent and telephone receipts in the absence of some compelling medical problem? For a time, new regulations required revealing the name of the father so he could be dunned for support. The prospect of abuse and battering resulting from such disclosures deterred some pregnant women from seeking certification; prenatal visitations occurred later rather than earlier in pregnancy.

Reagan policy beginning in 1982 imposed new penalties on the states for erroneous Medicaid enrollments in excess of 3%. More examiners were hired and certification review was made more stringent. Childbearing may be a sufficiently threatening experience to bring some pregnant women into the Medicaid examiner's office in order to assure admission to a hospital for delivery. Similar anxiety does not work for early prenatal care and routine preventive health services for children. The new eligibilities for children have not stimulated an increase in the utilization of preventive services.

Many years ago rumor circulated that Wilbur Cohen had predicted so much chaos for Medicaid that it would compel the nation to move quickly toward a program of universal compulsory national health insurance. He underestimated our capacity to endure chaos, if not for ourselves, then for poor women and their children.

Disjunction between Service Needs and Financing Approaches

Conventional medical care has much to recommend it for many people. But something more is needed for many children. As Schorr so appropriately documented, that "something more" need not solve every problem that invites attention.[8] Children can be helped—and are being helped the world over—without social upheaval that dislodges prevailing economic systems, equalizes income, disturbs the nation's existing social structures, or even drastically changes predominant systems of medical care. An adequate system of care for children, however, must assure universal participation in a set of basic services and must link these services to psychosocial supports. A vision of improved access that leaves open a door is not sufficient. Neither is item-by-item financing that rarely covers the "soft" services judged by most analysts to be an essential part of necessary care. Capitation payments for managed care (e.g., HMOs) show very little more promise, as their programs are formulated around the needs of middle-class families who enjoy employment benefits.

Up-front financing is required to ensure outreach efforts and linkages to comprehensive programs of care. The provision of community health services is not a part of current efforts to expand health care financing. No evidence suggests that expanded Medicaid coverage promotes expansion of community services, except possibly for nursing homes, an unhappy parallel for the needs of children.

A Preventive Emphasis

The United States is unique among industrialized nations in attempting to integrate preventive health care into primary practice settings that are equipped and staffed for ambulatory curative care and that preserve a prerogative to decline to provide services to selected people. The attempt to integrate preventive and curative care not only monopolizes resources but fails to reach many people. Office-based physicians spend 50% to 75% of their time during well-child visits doing routine physical examinations—a laying on of hands of dubious benefit.[2] In general, physicians do not spend much time on preventive care. One study of the well-child visits to 23 pediatricians found that anticipatory guidance consumed only 8.4% of the average visit,[7] amounting to 97 seconds of anticipatory guidance for patients younger than 5 months and 7 seconds for 13- to 18-year-olds.[2]

Attempting to integrate routine preventive care into primary practice settings works to the disadvantage of poor people, many of whom are excluded from private offices. Other drawbacks include having expensive physician providers, rather than aides, nurses, or midwives, perform routine procedures. At the same time, complex sociomedical problems that might be revealed during routine visits may be ignored or brushed aside because the talents of social workers, nutritionists, psychologists, and home visitors cannot be marshalled except through complex referral systems.

Other countries rely on neighborhood, often school-based, public health clinics to ensure participation in routine preventive care, parallel to and interactive with the network of practitioners, hospitals, and other providers who serve children when they are ill or indisposed. Such a system exists in some places in the United States, but it is not integral to national health policy.

The Lack of Funds

The most troublesome obstacle in the way of progress toward an enlightened health policy for children is the national debt. Even as popular sentiment grows that new public initiatives are required, our capacity to finance them is seriously constrained by an annual deficit of $150 billion and a requirement to achieve a balanced budget by 1993. The Reagan ideology against social spending has been implemented by a strategy that spends 28% of the federal budget on the military establishment, accumulating a debt burden that seems to foreclose other initiatives. Breaking the stalemate will require increased taxes, which most analysts advocate and all politicians deny, and recognition that enormous military expenditures fail to protect national security in some substantial ways. The health, vigor, and potential for productivity of young people, perhaps for the next generation, have been traded off in favor of an expensive military presence on every continent. We are reported to have more troops in Korea now than during the Korean War; we defend European countries in a way that enables them to spend a proportion of their own budgets on defense at levels less than half our own. Without reverting to an isolationist stance, the improved health of American children would benefit from a perspective that increasingly relies on diplomatic and economic means to maintain international harmony. This view is widely denigrated as dangerously unpatriotic. The most substantial Reagan legacy has been the shaping of American values into a Rambo mentality. The first condition to improve child health may be to overcome that mind-set.

A Vision for the Future

A vision of remedies and solutions to develop a health care system for children features three initiatives, none of which are alien to our national traditions.

The first initiative would establish a national health care financing system that might be age-specific but which must be universal, possibly in the fashion of Medicare. The means-tested reimbursement (Medicaid), which is linked to welfare payments and welfare agencies and which allows extensive state variation on the scope of implementation, should be discontinued.

The second initiative would institutionalize standards that include both outcome and selected process measures into all publicly financed systems of health care. The standards, drawing on experience with the 1990 Objectives for the Nation[6] and the Model Standards for Community Preventive Health Services,[3] should be incorporated into block grants and into contracts that involve payment of federal funds to insurance companies and major providers of health care. We have a long history of expressed dissatisfaction with the status of children's health. The means are now available for defining precisely what we hope to achieve and for controlling the means by which those expectations can be met. The serious adoption of even a few outcome standards might have a profound effect on achieving greater equity of care and rationalizing resource allocation.

The third initiative would require dramatically strengthening the public health infrastructure, operative at local levels, with the capacity to monitor children's health trends and the means to intervene with appropriate services rendered either directly or under contract with other providers. The infrastructure would require federal financing with standards and accountability consistently implemented between the federal government and the various state health agencies. Direct federal health service operations at community levels would be reserved for and would be invoked wherever problems are so severe that they do not yield to state action or where a state is persistently delinquent in complying with national standards of care.

All of these measures could be undertaken now; there are ample precedents for each of them. The timetable for their implementation invites debate between social activists and incrementalists. In resolving that debate, some limits are required. If we move incrementally, all three initiatives must be advanced concurrently. Temptations will be strong to expand financing, a little at a time, as we are doing now with Medicaid, and to leave for a later day the troublesome issues of enforcing standards and of assuring participation in essential services through the action of public agencies. Increased financing is essential, but without the other initiatives, it may move us further toward disaster. More money for business as usual, without safeguards that ensure participation in a defined set of essential services, will enrich the wrong priorities and will entrench present inequities.

People may ask if this vision does not rely excessively on the weakest part of our health care system—the public health sector. Skeptics should look carefully at the best public models, as we tend to look to the best private models. The best public health agencies are commendable, and they are replicable. Our present problems derive in large part because we have starved public health agencies, while lavishly financing every other part of the health care system.

Strong public health services are not the entire answer to improved health for children, however; income transfers, housing, day care, supervised recreation, family planning, and sexuality education are all legitimate and desirable approaches. But every feasible approach must include, if it is to be successful, a strong public health component.

Evidence has been marshalled to confirm that children have suffered under changes operative since passage of the Omnibus Budget Reconciliation Act of 1981. But not all changes were retrogressive, and not all prospects are gloomy. Many states and local jurisdictions have responded to recent adversities with inspired innovation and a new sense of mission to identify and serve neglected populations. These efforts have been weakened by inadequate financing and by uneven exercise of local initiative, which has not been supported, informed, or regulated by a sense of national purpose. A way is open to improve these circumstances by strengthening the role of the federal government in matters of health policy and financing. The federal role probably cannot revert, except in extraordinary circumstances, to a posture of direct participation in community services in the fashion of the 1960s. Greater promise is possible through expanding the federal role to finance, set standards for, and monitor the work of states and local jurisdictions in achieving mutually established health status objectives. In that endeavor, the recent work of many agencies attempting to refine the policy relevant understanding of health status measures will be critical.

References

1. Anderson OW. Health care: can there be equity? United States, Sweden and England. New York: John Wiley and Son, 1972.

2. Charney E. Well child care as axiom. Well Child Care. Columbus, OH: Ross Roundtable, 1986.

3. Centers for Disease Control. Model standards: a guide for community preventive health services. Washington, DC: American Public Health Association, 1985.

4. Enthoven A. Managed competition: an agenda for action. Health Affairs 1988;7:26.

5. Fuchs V. The "competitive revolution" in health care. Health Affairs 1988;7:5.

6. Public Health Service. Promoting health/preventing disease: objectives for the nation. Washington, DC: U.S. Government Printing Office, 1980.

7. Reisinger K, Bires J. Anticipatory guidance in pediatric practice. Pediatrics 1980;66:889.

8. Schorr L. Within our reach: breaking the cycle of disadvantage. New York: Anchor Doubleday, 1988.

9. Starr P. The social transformation of American medicine. New York: Basic Books, 1982.

10. U.S. General Accounting Office. Prenatal Care. Medicaid Recipients and Uninsured Women Obtain Insufficient Care. GAO-HRD-87-137. Washington, DC: GAO, 1987.